Praise for *The Five*

"What a treasure to find this book, which provides the best guide to Traditional Chinese Medicine I have ever read!"
—Ann Louise Gittleman, *New York Times* bestselling author of more than 35 books on health and nutrition

"A beautifully illustrated book that brings Chinese medicine to life. It is a wonderful handbook packed with practical suggestions of how to stay healthy."
—Bill Manahan, MD, past president, American Holistic Medical Association

"Warren King has created a masterful work that introduces the concept of the five Chinese elements to readers who may know nothing about them as well as those who are very familiar with them. His explanations of each element are clear, informative, and beautifully illustrated. Warren also provides the blunt truth about the food we eat and helpful measures on how we can take our health back. This is a must-read for anyone who is on the path to getting healthy."
—Carole Hyder, author of *Wind and Water: Your Personal Feng Shui Journey*

"The Five Elements of Healing *not only teaches you the language of your body but literally invites you to dance with your body. The text itself dances along with poetry and art.* The Five Elements of Healing *reaches so far beyond the organs themselves. It engages every aspect of your being, your senses, inner child and soul. This is definitely a book you will want to purchase and make part of your healing library!"*
—Cathryn Taylor, MA, MFT, LADC, author of *The Inner Child Workbook*

THE FIVE
ELEMENTS OF
Healing

THE FIVE ELEMENTS OF

Healing

木 火 土 全 水

A Practical Guide to Making Sense of Your Symptoms

WARREN KING

Lanto Press

For information, address:

Lanto Press
Los Angeles, CA
Email: info@LantoPress.com

Library of Congress Control Number: 2019913957

ISBN: 978-1-936965-06-9

This publication may contain open source content. Although the author has made every reasonable attempt to achieve complete accuracy of the content, no responsibility is assumed for errors or omissions. Any trademarks, service marks, or copyrights are assumed to be the property of their respective owners and are used only for reference. There is no implied endorsement in the use of any of them.

Cover design by Nita Ybarra
Composition and layout by Connie Kroskin
Original artwork as noted by Paivi King and Connie Kroskin

For bulk orders, contact: info@LantoPress.com

For foreign and translation rights, please contact:
Nigel J. Yorwerth, Yorwerth Associates, LLC
Email: nigel@PublishingCoaches.com

Medical Disclaimer: Information in this book is provided for educational purposes only and is not intended as a substitute for the advice provided by your physician or other health-care professional. You should not use the information in this book for diagnosing or treating a health problem or disease or for prescribing any medication or other treatment. You should always speak with your physician or other health-care professional before taking any medication or nutritional or herbal remedy or adopting any treatment for a health problem. If you have or suspect that you have a medical problem, promptly contact your health-care provider. Never disregard professional medical advice or delay in seeking professional advice because of something you have read in this book. Information and statements regarding health in this book are not intended to diagnose, treat, cure, or prevent any disease.

Contents

About the Elements   1

Earth   Spleen, Pancreas, and Stomach
Change of Season (Indian Summer)   9

Metal   Lung and Large Intestine
Autumn   31

Water   Kidney and Bladder
Winter   54

Wood   Liver and Gallbladder
Spring   78

Fire   Heart and Small Intestine
Summer   101

Five Elements Correspondence Chart   129
Five Elements Symptom Chart   130

Recipes to Heal Your Life with
the Five Elements   131

Timely Tips to Toxin-Proof Your Life   153

Imagine that you had 10 servants that had as their life mission to keep you happy and healthy. They would work for you, keep you feeling positive, throw out the garbage, and perform hundreds of other tasks. You do have these servants. They are the 10 main organs of your body.

In this book you will learn the language these organs use to communicate with you. Now your symptoms will make sense and you will understand what your organs have been trying to tell you.

Ancient Chinese healers discovered the forces of the universe and how the five basic energies or "elements" relate to our organs and our health. In this full-color book you will find many tools, such as facial diagnosis, acupressure, cooking, herbology, and qigong, that will help you on the road to regaining or maintaining your health. You will discover the amazing connection between each organ and specific emotions.

Warren King has been a licensed acupuncturist for 27 years and has treated more than ten thousand patients. He has developed his intuition to be able to communicate with the intelligence of the body and the energy of the organs. Now he combines the ancient healing wisdom of the East with the modern understanding of how our organs work and puts it all together in this book, a feast for the eyes and the mind.

The section "Timely Tips to Toxin-Proof Your Life" has been included due to the fact that modern toxins are affecting our health in ways that the ancient healers could never have anticipated.

About the Elements

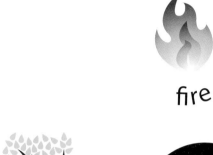

fire

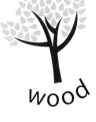

wood

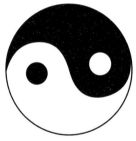

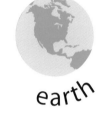

earth

water

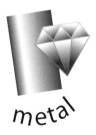

metal

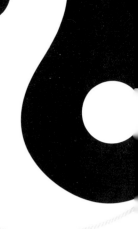

The Ancient Chinese

- They carefully observed nature.
- They noted the flow of energy in the universe.
- They applied this to an energy-based medicine.
- This medicine has practical use in healing the body and mind.

The Tai Chi or Yin / Yang

- Everything in existence has a polarity.
- There are dual energies within the circle of the one wholeness, the Tao.
- We call them yin and yang.

Everything Has Polarity

- Expansive and contractive
- Hot and cold
- Light and dark
- Male and female
- Outside and inside
- Positive and negative

Yin within Yang, Yang within Yin

- Notice the dots within the two halves.

- Nothing is absolute; within yin there is yang, and yang within yin.

- When something goes to the extreme it turns into its opposite.

  When you inhale all the way, you must exhale.
  When you exhale all the way, you must inhale.

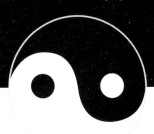

There is a flow of energy in the universe, and if you go with the current it can be fun. You can try the sidestroke or the backstroke. But if you go against the flow, it's hard work. You get illness and have no energy for psychological and spiritual development.

Try to understand life as energy. In physics, matter is not thought of as solid but as condensed energy. That energy has two types: expansive and contractive. Your heart and lungs and cells are continuously expanding and contracting.

Stress is yang and tightening, so some people reach for alcohol, which is yin and expansive. See if you can find better ways to achieve the balance your body is seeking. **We have to experiment on ourselves to find out how to balance these energies.**

3

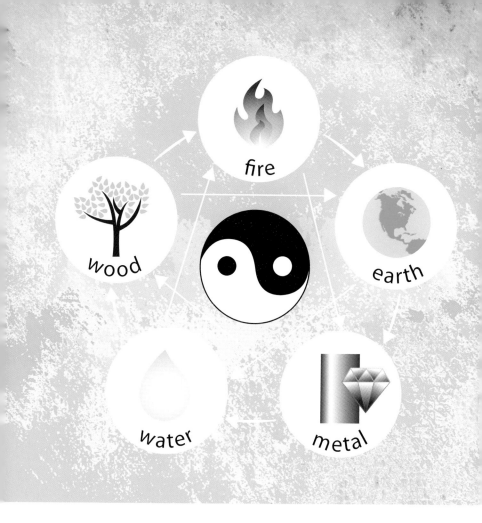

The Five Elements

- Yin and yang can be broken into five parts.
- They are often called the elements.
- They can be called the five phases of energy.
- The movement of energy from expansion to contraction, and from contraction to expansion.

Cycling of the Five Elements

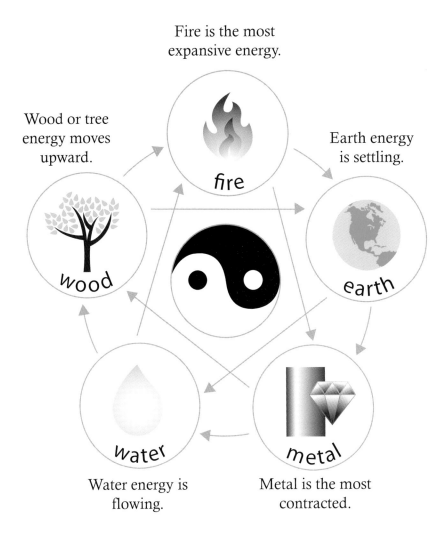

Fire is the most expansive energy.

Wood or tree energy moves upward.

Earth energy is settling.

fire

wood

earth

water

metal

Water energy is flowing.

Metal is the most contracted.

Five Elements and Health

- The Chinese applied the five elements to the body.

- This became the basis of Oriental medicine.

- There is a yin/yang organ pair for each element.

- One organ is usually solid, and the paired organ is hollow.

"Uplifting" ©2018 Connie Kroskin

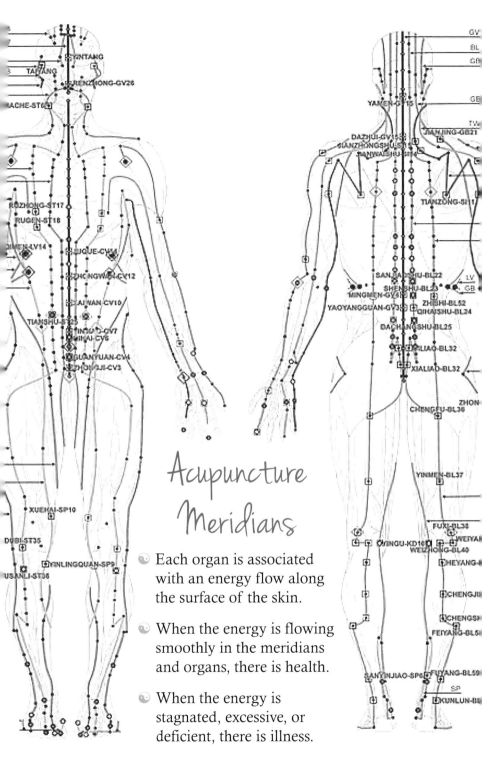

Acupuncture Meridians

- Each organ is associated with an energy flow along the surface of the skin.

- When the energy is flowing smoothly in the meridians and organs, there is health.

- When the energy is stagnated, excessive, or deficient, there is illness.

Modifying Energy Flow

The energy flow can be manipulated by various means.

- Acupuncture needles

- Acupressure

- Heat (moxibustion)

- Suction with cupping

- Modern methods such as electricity, crystals or gems, infrared heat, magnetism, or lasers

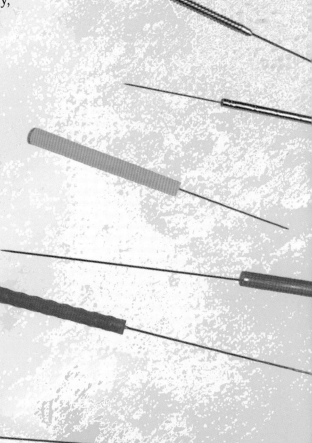

The Earth Element
Spleen, Pancreas, and Stomach

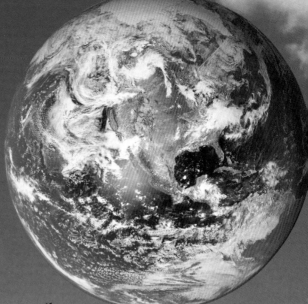

Earth

The acrid scent of compost pile
The diaper of a newborn child
Earth, just turned, in garden bed
The roses of the newly wed
The freshest air, when storm has passed
The fragrance of the fresh cut grass
I bring the fire of life to form
Your soul with flesh I do adorn
Between the seasons I give you rest
Truly I am the cosmic breast
I would not have you burn your lips
You must have reality in tiny sips
A handful of dirt that teems with life
If you like, I am spirit's wife
In volcanic ash new life shall creep
Pollen sprouting to pistil's deep
The softness of each petal rare
Floral fragrance distilled with care
My joy to serve, as farmer's toil
All you need springs from my soil.

—Warren King

Energy of Earth

Think of it as energy settling down

When the fire has passed its peak and ashes form, creating earth.

Energy is moving downward, coalescing, like the formation of compost

Like water coming down as rain.

Earth in the Daily Cycle

🌀 Because earth energy is downward, it has to do with afternoon, so earth rules the energy of afternoon.

🌀 Do you feel your energy drop in the afternoon? That is due to a blood sugar drop, which is related to the pancreas or spleen in Eastern medicine.

Earth in the Yearly Cycle

🌀 Indian summer is like the afternoon of the year.

🌀 Not quite summer, but not quite fall.

🌀 Earth is also seen as the cycle of transition between every season.

Earth Element Organs

Earth corresponds to the spleen and pancreas.

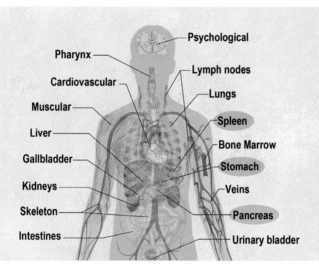

Pharynx
Cardiovascular
Muscular
Liver
Gallbladder
Kidneys
Skeleton
Intestines

Psychological
Lymph nodes
Lungs
Spleen
Bone Marrow
Stomach
Veins
Pancreas
Urinary bladder

The spleen acts as a filter against foreign organisms that infect the bloodstream. It also filters out old red blood cells from the bloodstream and decomposes them.

The spleen also acts as a blood reservoir. It manufactures red blood cells at the end of fetal development.

The pancreas is yellowish, seven inches long, and is behind the stomach. It releases three digestive enzymes into the small intestine to break down carbohydrates, proteins, and fats.

The islets of Langerhans, a region within the pancreas, secrete two hormones, insulin and glucagon. Insulin lowers the blood sugar level and increases the amount of glycogen (stored carbohydrate) in the liver; glucagon has the opposite action.

When the cells stop producing insulin, you have diabetes. When cells stop responding to insulin, you have insulin resistance.

Paired Organ of Earth

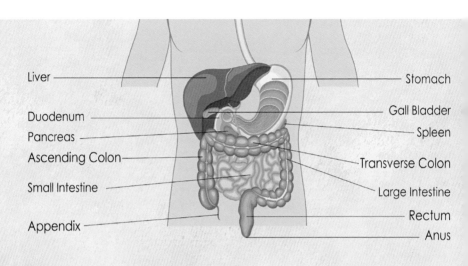

Liver — Stomach
Duodenum — Gall Bladder
Pancreas — Spleen
Ascending Colon — Transverse Colon
Small Intestine — Large Intestine
Appendix — Rectum
— Anus

The stomach is about 12 inches long and 6 inches wide at its widest point. Its capacity is about one quart in an adult.

The surface of the mucosa is honeycombed with over 35,000 gastric glands that secrete hydrochloric acid. The stomach churns the food, but proper chewing, which mixes the food with saliva, begins digestion of starches and is needed to make the particles small enough for proper digestion.

Blood sugar problems are not all from sugar but are also from fat. High fat content in blood dulls insulin's effectiveness. Overweight people are more likely to become diabetic. Most people of average weight are less likely to become diabetic.

Fats tighten the pancreas so that it becomes less effective. French fries, greasy foods, and heavy animal fats can lead to blood sugar problems. Ice-cold foods and drinks shock the stomach and pancreas. Americans consume ice-cold water and ice cream all year round, even in winter.

Body Part Association

Each organ is associated with, or considered to rule, a certain body part and sense organ. **The spleen rules the muscles.**

The spleen is connected to the pancreas, and one symptom of diabetes is wasting of the muscles.

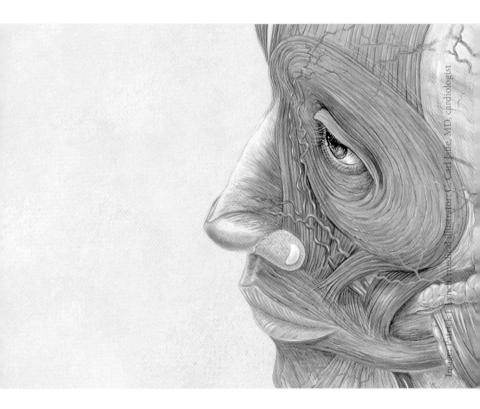

Image: Patient5 | Photo credit: medical illustrator, C. Carl Jaffe, MD, cardiologist

Sense Organ Association

The spleen corresponds to the mouth and lips.

Cold sores on the lips can be associated with a spleen imbalance.

The Taste of Earth

The flavor associated with the spleen,
pancreas, and stomach is sweet.

No flavor causes more problems than sweet. It's like a drug
that people want to get off of, can go months without, then go
to a family gathering, try some, and suddenly need it daily.

Complex carbohydrates give strength, but simple sugars should
be kept to a minimum. They rob the body of B vitamins, disturb
mineral balance, rot teeth, and make the body tissues acid.

Blood sugar constantly fluctuates. When it's down, we crave
sweet. Eating a candy bar is like throwing gasoline on a fire;
you get a quick kick but have nothing left afterwards.

When your blood sugar is low, you can try a more complex
sweetener like rice syrup or barley malt. If you need a quick
sugar, you can try a tropical fruit.

**The long-term solution is to add sweet vegetables to
your diet: carrots, parsnips, rutabagas, squash, yams,
sweet potatoes, and other good, complex sugars.**

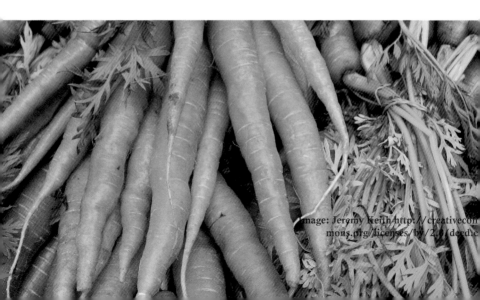

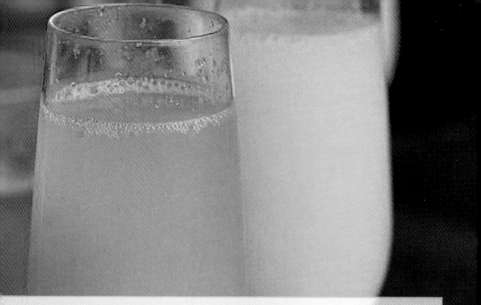

Fiber slows absorption, so if you need sugar faster you can have vegetable juice or fruit juice. Also if you have low blood sugar like hypoglycemia, whole grains are good. If you want to raise it faster, have some bread.

A sweet vegetable drink is a great home remedy to help with blood sugar imbalances. Drinking a broth made from sweet vegetables also alkalizes the body, balancing an excess acid state.

When you have a heavy meal you'll want something yin, sweet, and light after to balance it, so have some cooked berries or applesauce. If you have something more yang with heavy stuff like baked flour and oils, you'll still feel heavy and continue craving sweets.

The purpose of dessert is to be light, not heavy. Sluggish, overweight individuals or those with dampness, such as excess mucus, should take sweets very sparingly, and even whole food carbohydrates moderately. Chewing carbohydrates well makes them less mucus forming.

Spleen / Pancreas and Sweets

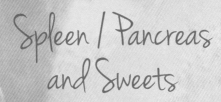

- When sugar enters the system, the pancreas secretes insulin to open the cells to the sugar.

- Artificial sweeteners can cause diabetes by throwing off the balance of bacteria in the intestines.

- Complex carbohydrates break down more slowly in the system, creating less of a blood sugar spike, and therefore, less of an emotional roller coaster.

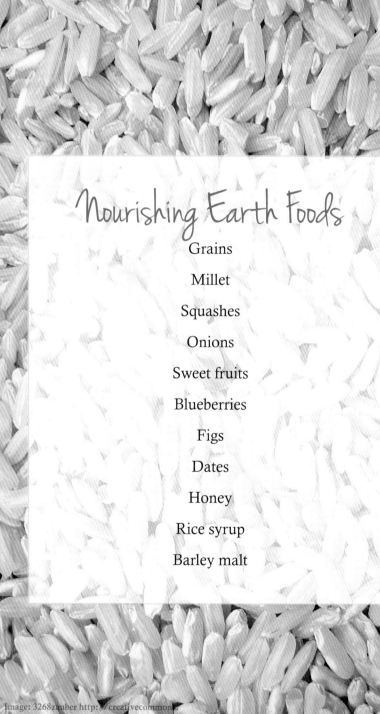

Nourishing Earth Foods

Grains

Millet

Squashes

Onions

Sweet fruits

Blueberries

Figs

Dates

Honey

Rice syrup

Barley malt

Cooking Styles

Roasting

Stewing

Beating

Mashing

Purees

Jams & Jellies

Desserts

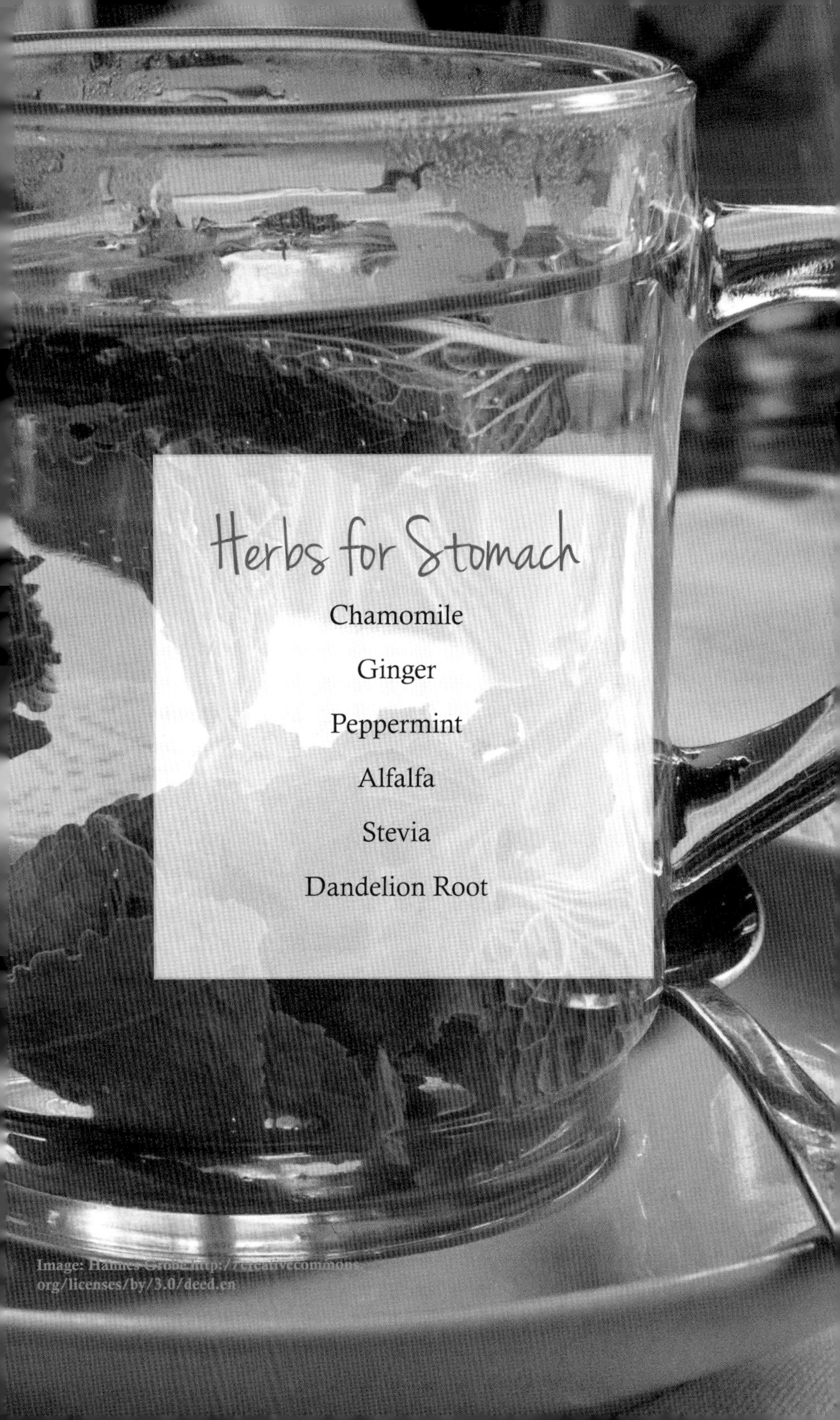

Herbs for Stomach

Chamomile

Ginger

Peppermint

Alfalfa

Stevia

Dandelion Root

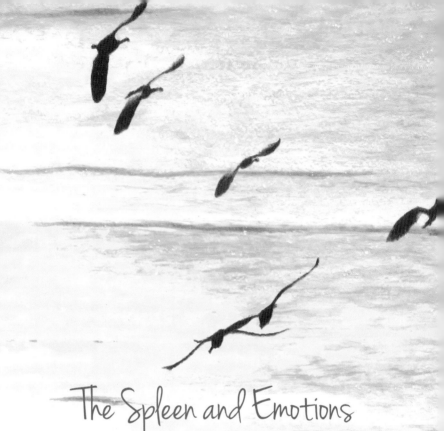

The Spleen and Emotions

- Thought, mental function, and concentration have to do with the spleen.

- Empathy, understanding, and compassion are signs of a balanced earth element.

- An imbalanced earth element can produce overthinking and worry.

If the spleen is out of balance you feel anxious, worried, and too sympathetic or sensitive.

When in balance you feel calm, soothed, more discriminating and self-determined. You feel like singing.

When you have a healthy stomach, it results in mental and emotional stability, while imbalance leads to worry, skepticism, and anxiety.

"Golden Glide" ©2018 Connie Kroskin

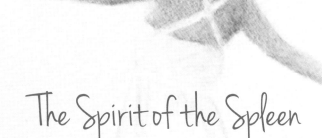

The Spirit of the Spleen

- The spirit that incarnates in the spleen is called the Yi.

- The Yi has to do with intention, purpose, clarity of thought, altruism, and integrity.

- Chronic worrying and rumination are signs of an imbalanced Yi.

The Yi represents the power of the earth in us. It is the spirit that gives us the capacity for sustained intention, purpose, clarity of thought, altruism, and integrity. It is related to the emotions of sympathy and the organ of the spleen.

It supports our capacity for thought, intention, reflection, and the act of applying ourselves to our heart's purpose.

It gives us the ability to concentrate, study, and memorize data for one's work, and endows us with the capacity for clear thought. **In other words, it allows us to apply our spirit to the world of form.**

"Planes Woman" ©2018 Connie Kroskin

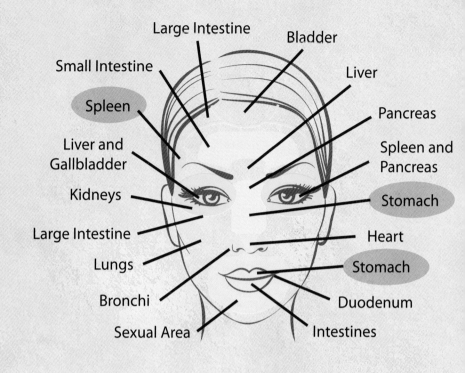

Large Intestine
Bladder
Small Intestine
Liver
Spleen
Pancreas
Liver and Gallbladder
Spleen and Pancreas
Kidneys
Stomach
Large Intestine
Heart
Lungs
Stomach
Bronchi
Duodenum
Sexual Area
Intestines

Facial Diagnosis

- **The face never lies.**

- The bridge of the nose is the stomach.

- The eyelids reflect the state of the spleen.

The stomach is reflected in the upper lip and bridge of the nose. A swollen upper lip is caused by refined carbohydrates, fruit, alcohol, or white flour.

A contracted stomach can be seen in a tight upper lip and can be from meat, eggs, salt, dry baked food, or fasting. Blood vessels expanded on the eyelids or styes can indicate a spleen imbalance.

The Spleen Meridian

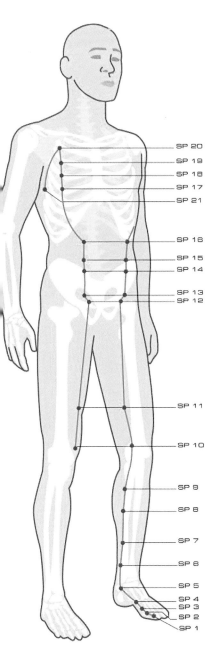

SP 20
SP 19
SP 18
SP 17
SP 21
SP 16
SP 15
SP 14
SP 13
SP 12
SP 11
SP 10
SP 9
SP 8
SP 7
SP 6
SP 5
SP 4
SP 3
SP 2
SP 1

- From outside of big toe to chest.

- 21 acupuncture points.

- The spleen governs the transportation and transformation of nutrients, helping food become qi, or life force energy, and blood.

- It has to do with digestion, and a dysfunction leads to bloating, diarrhea, and lack of appetite.

Some problems related to the spleen meridian can be big toe issues, inner knee pain, swelling of the inner leg, diaphragm issues, and esophagus or tongue symptoms.

Internal pathway blockages can create diaphragm and lung conditions, tightness in the chest, feeling of something in the throat (plum pit), and eye pain.

Stomach Meridian

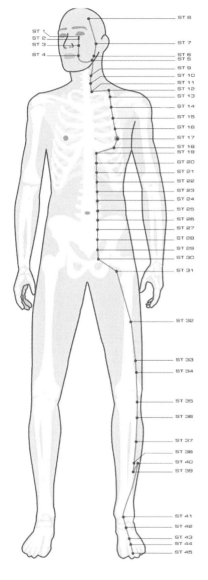

- From the eye to the second toe.

- 45 acupuncture points.

- The stomach initiates the metabolism of food and drink.

Second and third toe are the end of the stomach meridian. If they are longer than the big toe and webbed, this indicates excess fruit, sugar, medications, or refined foods during pregnancy, giving an expanded, or yin, stomach.

If these two toes are much shorter than the big toe or bend toward the big toe, your mother may have eaten too much salt or animal food during pregnancy.

Vigorous massage of these two toes helps nausea or stomach upset.

Meridian imbalances can create cheek marks, throat issues, breast issues, digestive and ovarian issues, pain or skin issues on area of the legs where the meridian runs, knee pain, and acid reflux or frequent hunger.

Spleen Acupoint

Spleen 6-Sanyinjiao-three yin junction
(Liver, kidney, and spleen channels meet at
this point.)

Location: Put four fingers together and
measure this length above the inner ankle
bone, point is located just behind the bone
(tibia).

Benefits: Poor digestion, insomnia,
anemia, water retention, menstrual or
female organ problems, calms the spirit.

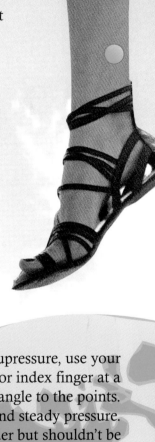

For acupressure, use your
middle or index finger at a
90-degree angle to the points.
Apply firm and steady pressure.
This may be tender but shouldn't be
painful. Hold the point for about three
minutes. You can also visualize light
coming out of your finger and illuminating
the meridian and the associated organ.

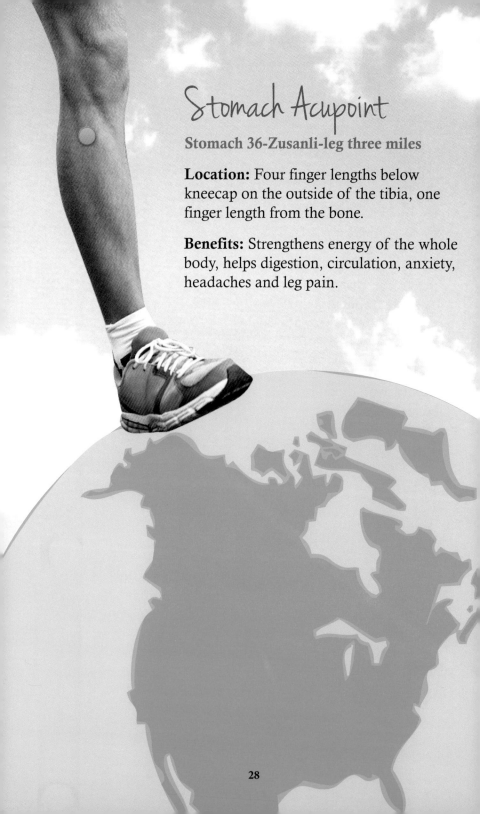

Stomach Acupoint

Stomach 36-Zusanli-leg three miles

Location: Four finger lengths below kneecap on the outside of the tibia, one finger length from the bone.

Benefits: Strengthens energy of the whole body, helps digestion, circulation, anxiety, headaches and leg pain.

Time of Day Earth Meridians Peak

Energy peaks in the spleen channel at 9 to 11 AM.

Energy peaks in the stomach channel at 7 to 9 AM.

Energy travels in the acupuncture organs and meridians throughout the day in a 24-hour period.

It is interesting that we should be eating and digesting breakfast in the peak times for the stomach and spleen. Research is really showing how eating a good breakfast is a key for weight and blood sugar and for learning, all earth element issues.

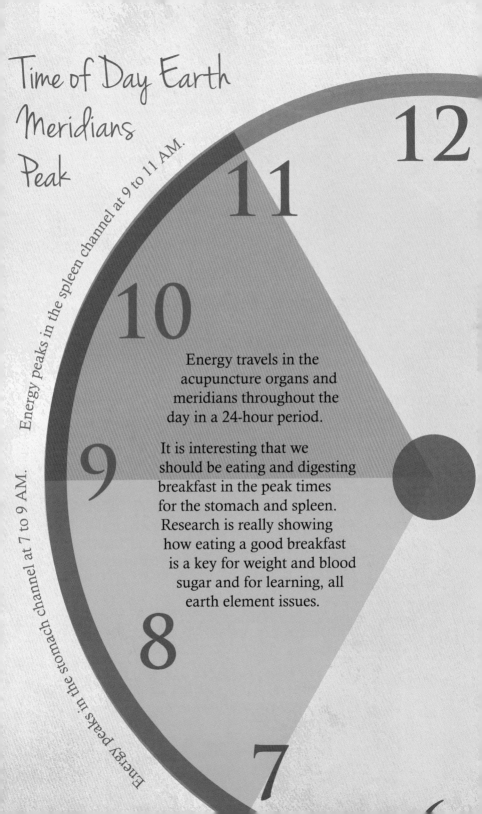

Healing Sound for the Spleen

Qigong has a healing sound for the major organs, *Hu* is the sound for the spleen (*whooo*).

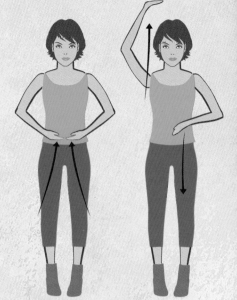

STEP 1: Stand naturally upright. Inhale and bring your hands next to your breast area with your palms facing up and fingers pointing at each other. During inhalation, imagine leading the energy from your big toe on your left foot up the inside of your left leg and up to your spleen.

STEP 2: Exhale and rotate your right palm out and up. Rotate your left palm in and down, then extend your right hand up and your left hand down. When exhaling, imagine leading impurities from your spleen out, passing a point at your left armpit, then down to a point just below the left rib cage. When exhaling, make the *Hu* sound. While drawing your stomach and the center of the perineum in and up, squeeze out the impurities from your spleen.

STEP 3: Inhale and bring both hands down facing each other like in step 1. Next, rotate your left palm out and up then rotate your right palm in and down. Next, extend your left palm up and your right palm down. Exhale as you did on the other side. During inhalation, imagine leading the energy from your left big toe up the inside of your left leg and up to your spleen. Repeat a total of six inhalations and exhalations.

The Metal Element
Lung and Large Intestine

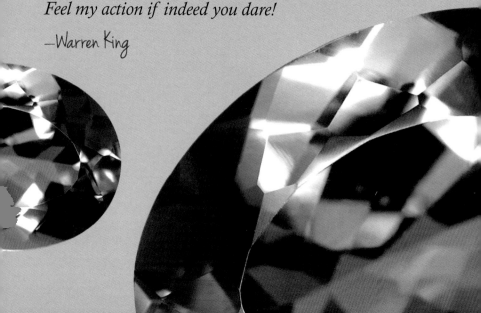

Metal

Those on earth call me real
No phantasm or cloud with me you'll feel
Hit your thumb with a hammer, bang!
I am the essence who is most yang
Those of the East named me metal
Perhaps the new age shall call me crystal
Strength and tension, pressure and strain
The bone of form, the skull for your brain
God's kingdom extended to the realms most dense
Valiant souls then journeyed hence
The fist of the victor, the diamond, the will
The spine of a cactus, an avalanche spill
To air I am thunder, to water I'm hail
My iron stokes fires, to wood I'm the nail
To earth I'm the shovel, I'm the essence of men
The bullet, the sword blade, the tip of the pen
The teeth of the lion, the nails of a hare
Feel my action if indeed you dare!

—Warren King

Energy of Metal

Don't think of it as a piece of metal.

Think of it more like the most contracted energy.

It could be metal or a stone or a crystal

...or water freezing into ice.

Metal in the Daily Cycle

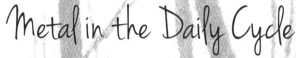

▽ Since metal is downward energy, it has to do with the sunset.

▽ So metal rules the energy of evening.

▽ Think of how you start going within at dusk.

▽ Do you feel like crashing after work?

Metal in the Yearly Cycle

▽ Fall is like the sunset of the year.

▽ Everything is moving inward and downward.

▽ If you feel worse in the fall with allergies, for example, you could be experiencing a metal imbalance.

Metal Element Organs

Metal corresponds to the lungs.

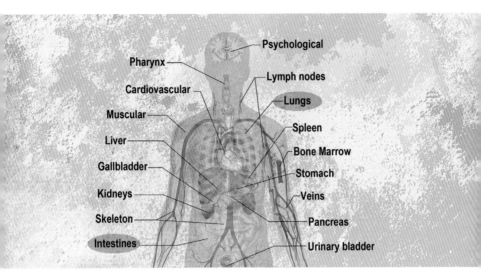

- Psychological
- Pharynx
- Lymph nodes
- Cardiovascular
- Lungs
- Muscular
- Spleen
- Liver
- Bone Marrow
- Gallbladder
- Stomach
- Kidneys
- Veins
- Skeleton
- Pancreas
- Intestines
- Urinary bladder

▼ At rest, a person breathes about 14 to 16 times per minute. During exercise it could increase to over 60 times per minute.

▼ New babies at rest breathe between 40 and 50 times per minute. By age 5 it decreases to around 25 times per minute.

▼ The total surface area of the alveoli (tiny air sacs in the lungs) is the size of a tennis court.

▼ The lungs are the only organ in the body that can float on water.

Paired Organ of Metal

The hollow organ paired with the lungs is the large intestine

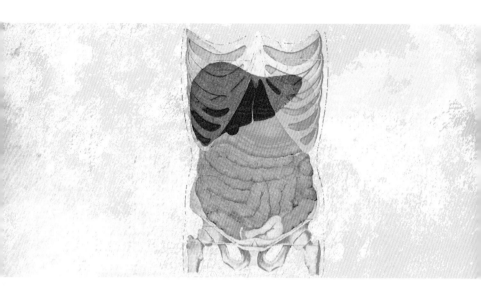

- ▼ The large intestine is about five feet long. The appendix hangs off the large intestine, and scientists are only beginning to understand that it is a reservoir for the beneficial flora in the large intestine.

- ▼ We have as many bacteria in our large intestine as cells in our bodies, about 75 trillion, and over 400 species of micro-organisms.

- ▼ Water and some vitamins and minerals are reabsorbed from the waste that moves on to become stool.

- ▼ It can take food three days to move through the 15 feet of the gastrointestinal tract. In other cultures it can take four to six hours due to a better diet, more exercise, and less stress.

◆ About 70% of the cells that make up the body's immune system are found in the wall of the gut.

◆ When parasites or yeast (candida) overgrow in the intestines you can get systemic health problems.

◆ Intestinal problems are often the forerunner of other health problems and chronic constipation is a prewarning sign for cancer, especially for breasts, which are over the lungs and connected energetically with the large intestine.

Large Intestine Health Issues
- Crohn's disease
- Colitis
- Irritable bowel
- Gas
- Bloating
- Constipation
- Diarrhea
- Hemorrhoids
- Colon cancer
- Toxic intestines can create many skin conditions.
- Sinus problems are often associated with the intestines as well. Psoriasis and asthma often go together; when one is suppressed it may lead to the other.

Our intestines are overfed, overworked, and underexercised.

Image: Tatiane Brito

Body Part Association

Each organ is associated with, or considered to rule, a certain body part and sense organ. **Lungs rule the skin.**

Lungs have to do with what is called the wei chi or defensive energy of the body that surrounds the skin. Sweating is thought to be related to the lungs, so it is no surprise that those who take saunas in the winter have fewer colds. Many Chinese herb formulas for infections have diaphoretic herbs, or herbs that promote sweating. Thus the invading wind and cold are pushed outward so the infection doesn't go deeper.

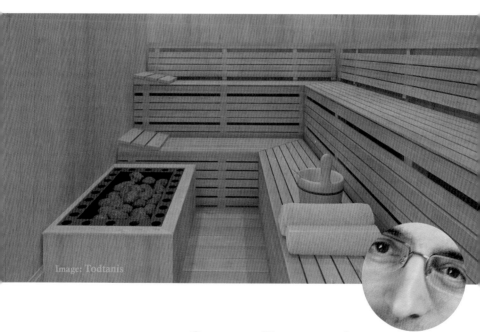

Image: Todtanis

Sense Organ Association

The lungs correspond to the nose.

The nose and sinuses are all considered part of the lung energy system.

The Taste of Metal

The flavor associated with the lungs
and large intestine is pungent.

Pungent
flavors, like
ginger, are
very good
for digestion.
This flavor
dispels
mucus from
the lungs
and large
intestine.

Nourishing Metal Foods

Onions	Leeks
Garlic	Chinese cabbage
Ginger	Bok choy
Daikon radish	Celery
Peppers	Cucumber
Red radishes	Spicy peppers
Chives	Rice

◆ Dairy can produce mucus, as can flour products like breads, cookies, cakes, and muffins. If you eat more than a moderate portion or don't chew well, your body will produce mucus and your food will not be properly digested.

Pungent foods clear mucus from the lungs, improve digestion, and expel gas from the intestines. They moisten the kidneys, affecting the fluids of the whole body. Thus they increase saliva and sweat.

◆ Whole grain bread can be healthy, but if you have mucus in the sinuses or lungs it's best to cut it out of your diet.

If you eat too many baked flour products, which are yang, they will slow digestion and produce mucus. To counterbalance this effect, add these vegetables, which are good-quality yin and balance out dairy as well.

◆ Metal foods stimulate blood circulation and tonify the heart. They clear obstructions and improve sluggish liver function.

Those who are dull, sluggish, lethargic, or too heavy, as well as those with dampness or mucus in the lungs and large intestine are benefited by pungent foods.

The vegetables listed above can help if you feel mentally unclear or unfocused.

Photograph: Hedwig Storch

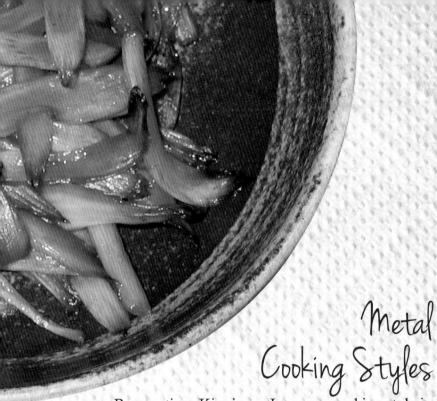

Metal Cooking Styles

Preparation: Kinpira, a Japanese cooking style in which matchstick-cut veggies are braised in oil, then water is added, and pressure-cooked.

Remember, metal is the most yang element. Dense root vegetables cut into little matchsticks is a very yang cutting style.

Pressure cooking in metal cookware and adding lots of inward pressure imparts a strong yang force. The opposite, and most yin type of cooking, is microwaving in which food is heated by exploding water molecules.

Pressure cooking grains such as rice, which is the grain for metal, and vegetables and beans makes them very soft and digestible, which soothes the mucous membranes of the lungs, sinuses, and large intestine.

Try cooking kinpira with carrots and burdock root, which is the most yang root there is. Burdock root can grow three feet long and can break rocks.

41

Photograph: Ryosuke Hosoi

Lungs / Large Intestine and Health

Often the lungs and sinuses reflect the condition of the large intestine.

Make sure that parasites, yeast, fungus, and bad bacteria are eliminated from the large intestine.

Fermented foods can help replenish the beneficial flora in the large intestine.

Examples are sauerkraut, kimchi, kombucha, yogurt, kefir, miso, and sourdough bread.

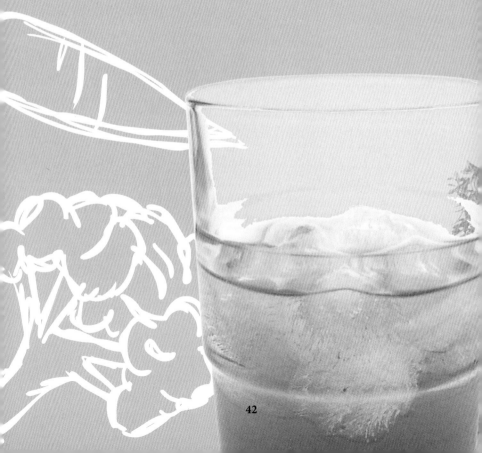

Herbs for Lungs

- Astragalus
- Fennel
- Goldenseal
- Licorice
- Thyme

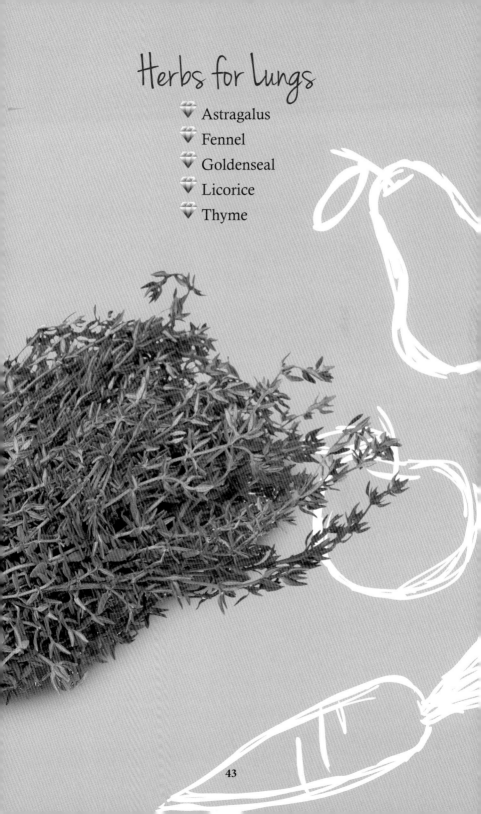

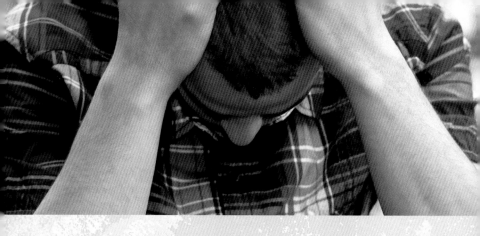

The Lungs/Large Intestine and Emotions

▼ The lungs are the seat of our feelings and sentiments, and allow us to feel sadness and grief.

▼ When the lungs are weak, one tends toward self-pity, quietude, inwardness, depression, lack of will and vitality, or antisocial behavior.

▼ When the lungs are hyperactive, one is more outwardly expressive of sadness and grief with crying, sobbing, verbal pessimism, or lashing out at others.

▼ Positive metal emotion includes discerning what is healthy and essential, and discerning what to take in and what to let go of.

It's interesting that lungs are the only organ we can directly control, and **crying and laughing are just strange ways of breathing.**

In the East, spirituality, meditation, and consciousness-raising involves control of the breath. So when lungs are an issue, you can feel lethargic and have difficulty thinking clearly. **When they are balanced, you feel more compassionate, energized, organized, and decisive.**

The Spirit of the Lungs

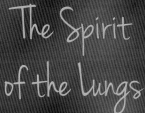

◆ The spirit that incarnates in the lungs is called the Po.

◆ The Po is our embodied knowing, our animal wit, our street smarts.

◆ It is closely related to the autonomic nervous system, the sensory receptors, especially the skin.

The Po is the part of us that can sniff out what's right or wrong, good or bad, safe or unsafe.

Deep below the level of our conscious ability to articulate in words what we think about a person, place, or situation, the Po spirit already knows, and whether or not we realize it, our body has begun to respond by contracting or expanding, hardening or softening.

Spending time with animals can help you tune into your Po, the animal soul within us.

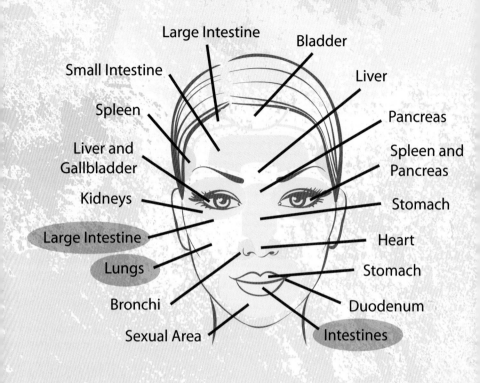

Large Intestine
Bladder
Small Intestine
Liver
Spleen
Pancreas
Liver and Gallbladder
Spleen and Pancreas
Kidneys
Stomach
Large Intestine
Heart
Lungs
Stomach
Bronchi
Duodenum
Sexual Area
Intestines

Facial Diagnosis

◈ **The face never lies.**

◈ The cheeks tell us about the condition of the lungs.

◈ The large intestine is reflected in the state of the lower lip.

Facial Diagnosis

Lungs are represented in the lower cheeks
at the level of the mouth.

Pimples: saturated animal fat, milk products, and sugar

White cheeks: milk products

Red: excess fruits, juices, stimulants, spices, sugar

Brown blotches: acid, mostly sugar, can be precancerous

Green: tendency toward cancer

Moles: animal protein

Beauty marks: past fever in the lungs

Swollen lower lip: refined carbohydrates, fruit, alcohol,
or white flour

Tight lower lip: contracted large intestine from meat,
eggs, salt, dry baked food, or fasting

The condition of the intestine can also be seen in the forehead,
with the small intestine in the middle and the large
intestine around the outside.

The Lung Meridian

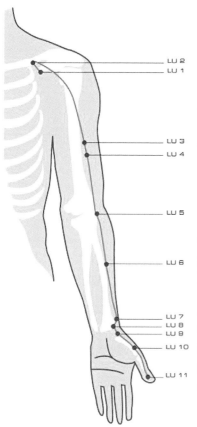

◆ From below the clavicle or collarbone, down inside of the arm to outside corner of the thumb.

◆ 11 acupuncture points.

◆ The lung governs respiration and the extraction of Qi from the air and plays a role in fluid metabolism.

Combines Qi of air with Qi of food and spreads it throughout body via meridians and blood.

Also distributes defensive or wei chi under the skin for protection against pathogens (our immunity), so sweating is an elimination and defense ruled by the lungs.

Lung Symptoms

shortness of breath

chest tightness

asthma

coughing

pain or skin issues along the meridian

pain in the thumbs or problems with the thumbnail

LU 2
LU 1
LU 3
LU 4
LU 5
LU 6
LU 7
LU 8
LU 9
LU 10
LU 11

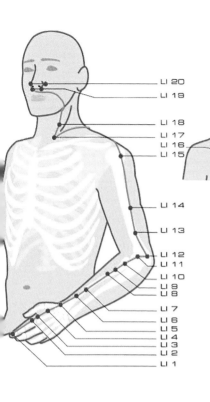

LI 20
LI 19
LI 18
LI 17
LI 16
LI 15
LI 14
LI 13
LI 12
LI 11
LI 10
LI 9
LI 8
LI 7
LI 6
LI 5
LI 4
LI 3
LI 2
LI 1

The Large Intestine Meridian

◆ From the index finger to the nose.

◆ 20 acupuncture points.

◆ The large intestine has to do with the absorption of water from food and excretion of feces.

Problems along the meridian can affect nose, lips and throat, shoulder, elbow, and wrist.

I treated a child who picked at his index fingernail until he made a hole right through it. It turned out that he had a parasite in his large intestine.

Now that you know that the large intestine rules the index finger, you can understand why nobody likes it pointed at them while being reprimanded!

Photograph: Dnalor 01 http://bit.ly/19NgZNS

Lung Acupoint

Lung 1-Zhongfu-Central Treasury

Location: Under the shoulder end of the collarbone, one hand width above the armpit, and one finger length inward.

Benefits: All lung problems, cough, asthma, congestion and phlegm. Skin problems, emotional tension, sore throat, shoulder and upper back pain.

For acupressure, use your mid or index finger at a 90-degree angle to the points. Apply firm and steady pressure, it may be tender but shouldn't be painful. Hold the point for about three minutes. You can also visualize light coming out of your finger and illuminating the meridian and the associated organ.

Large Intestine Acupoint

Large Intestine 4-Hegu-Joining of the Valleys

Location: In the web between the thumb and index finger on the back of the hand. At the highest point of the mound when these two digits are brought together.

Benefits: Allergies, sinus problems, headaches, itching, colds, and upper body.

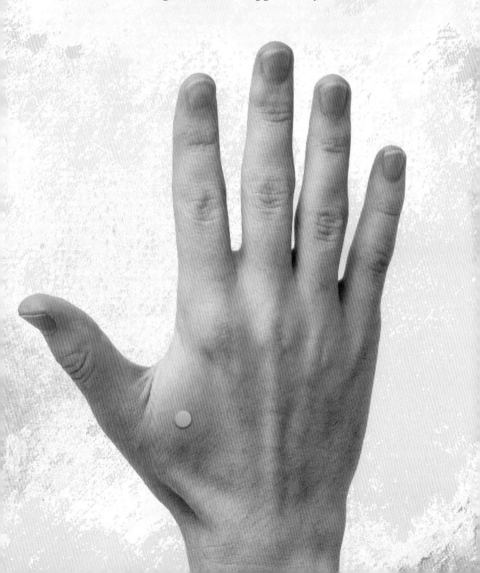

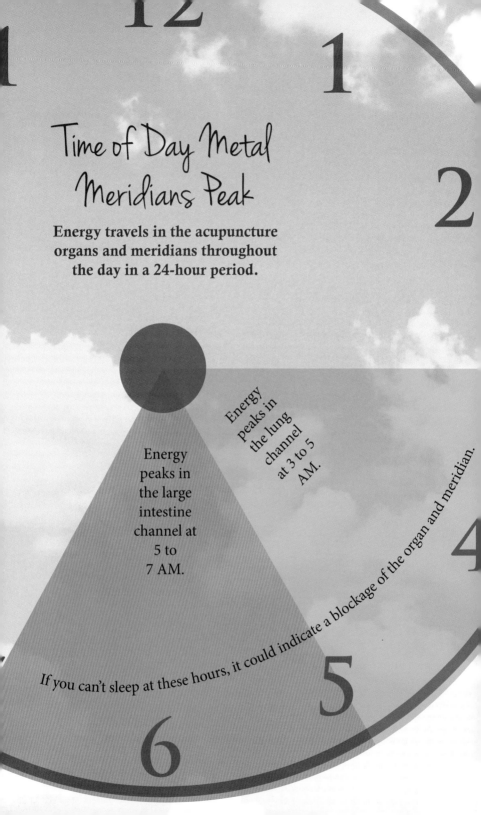

Time of Day Metal Meridians Peak

Energy travels in the acupuncture organs and meridians throughout the day in a 24-hour period.

Energy peaks in the lung channel at 3 to 5 AM.

Energy peaks in the large intestine channel at 5 to 7 AM.

If you can't sleep at these hours, it could indicate a blockage of the organ and meridian.

Healing Sound for the Lungs

Qigong has a healing sound for the major organs. *Si* is the sound for nourishing the lungs (*seeeee*).

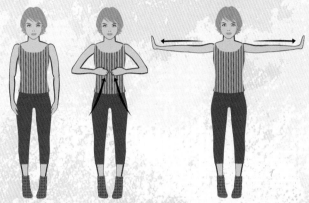

STEP 1: Stand or sit with your feet shoulder width apart, arms to your sides. Pay attention to your exhalation three times to remove the impurities from your lungs. Take a deep breath and imagine leading the energy (Qi) from the universe into your body, down to your second toe of your right foot.

STEP 2: Hold your breath. Raise your hands up in front of your body with your hands facing up and fingers pointing toward each other. When they reach the breast area, rotate your palms until they are facing out. As you raise your hands, imagine leading the energy from the second toe up the inside of your right leg and right front of your body into the lungs.

STEP 3: Exhale and begin making the *Si* (*seeeee*) sound. At the same time, push your arms to the sides as you hold up the center of the perineum and bring your abdomen in. As you make the *Si* sound, lead the impurities out of your lungs through your mouth and down the inside of your right arm going out of your thumbnail.

Repeat steps 1 to 3, six times.

The Water Element
Kidney and Bladder

Water

After such hard work, enjoy a shower
Though I am soft, I have no less power
My drops, through eons erode any rock
My nebulous vapor can rust any lock
I seek all places deep and low
I run not or jump, I relax and flow
I am the moist eyes of every daughter
To life I am mother, they know me as water
Lakes and oceans, rainstorm and dew
After the drought, all life I renew
Steam me, I'll condense, freeze me, I'll melt
I'm the flow of emotion, can't be known, just felt
I clean out all toxins, remove all debris
No one can live a moment without me
Hear me in song in the cry of the loon
Poets depict me in the face of the moon
Restrict my expression and soon you'll be old
Life is for living, water you can't hold
I love to dance in fountain and spring
In each beating heart, in each cell do I sing
My essence can fill the deepest hole
Feel now my presence thou precious soul.

—Warren King

Photograph: Henningklevjer http://bit.ly/1echp0B

Energy of Water

Imagine as water goes from ice
to flowing liquid water
before it vaporizes.

It has no form of its own and follows
the course of least resistance.

It seems weak, but it can carve the deepest
canyon and wear down the hardest rock.

"Blue Trees" ©2018 Connie Kroskin

Water in the Daily Cycle

💧 Water corresponds to nighttime.

💧 The time after sunset (metal) and before sunrise (wood).

💧 How is your night?

Night shift is called the graveyard shift for a reason. Kidneys recharge at night, so being awake at that time makes it hard to recharge your batteries.

Nighttime problems like insomnia or night sweats may be kidney related. So would tossing and turning in bed, grinding teeth at night, nightmares, bed-wetting or waking at night to urinate.

Water in the Yearly Cycle

💧 Water is connected with the winter.

💧 Nature goes within during winter.

💧 Winter is like the nighttime of the year.

Winter is cold. Not much is happening. Movement is slow, quiet, and still. Plants send their energy to the roots, animals slow down and some hibernate.

Kidneys like warmth and heat, so cold extremities are a sign of weak kidneys. Use of a ginger compress is a home remedy for weak kidneys. Sauna may benefit them as well.

Water Element Organs

Water corresponds to the solid organ of the kidneys.

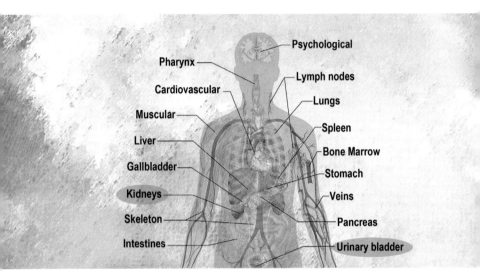

Each kidney is about five inches long and three inches wide. One of the main jobs is to filter waste out of your 1 to 1.5 gallons of blood as many as 400 times a day!

The kidneys also balance the volume of fluids and minerals in the body. They even make some of their own hormones, such as the one that tells the body to make red blood cells. The kidneys can also help regulate blood pressure.

The adrenal glands are associated with the kidneys and help protect against mental stress. In Chinese medicine kidneys are viewed as the center of the vital force or chi so it's important to keep them strong. They enable us to go out into life and handle problems.

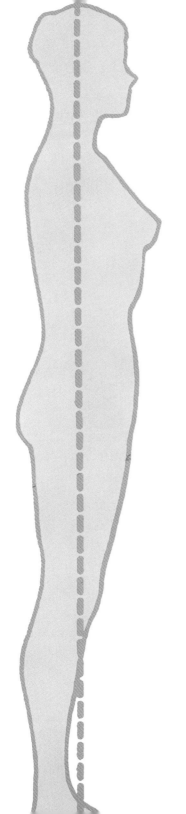

Salt can tighten kidneys and make them hold water. Too much protein can be hard on the kidneys. Meat is often a cause of kidney stones. Men need more protein than women and women need more oil than men.

The average person eats nine pounds of chemicals a year, a big stress on kidneys. Heavy metals such as mercury in silver fillings are an additional stressor.

Kidneys are often the underlying cause of arthritis.

Soft drinks high in phosphoric acid and sugar are hard on kidneys.

Kidneys rule sexual energy, so people on Viagra® and similar drugs really need to strengthen the kidneys.

If the kidneys are hard or calloused there can be fatty deposits or stones in the kidneys.

Kidneys can affect posture. Leaning forward can mean kidneys are too tight, and leaning backward when walking, sitting, and standing can indicate overly expanded kidneys.

Paired Organ of Water

The hollow paired organ of the kidneys
is the urinary bladder.

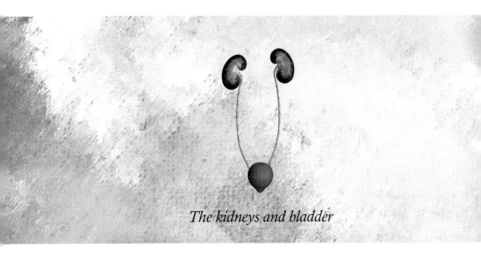

The kidneys and bladder

The bladder is a
storage sac that
holds the urine.
When the bladder
is about halfway
full, your body tells
you to urinate.

The bladder is such
a simple organ
that scientists are
beginning to be
able to grow them
in a lab.

Your Constitution

It is thought that our inherited energy, or Jing, is stored in our kidneys. **It is like a battery that we run on for the rest of our life, and it is not easy to recharge it once it has run down.**

Your constitution is what you are born with. But your condition is how you are now. So if you are born with a strong constitution but sleep little, play hard, take drugs, smoke or use alcohol excessively, eat too much, or are consumed with worry and frustration, you could have a shorter life. Likewise, if you inherited a weak constitution, but eat very cleanly, sleep long enough, exercise, and meditate, you could have a longer life.

Those with stronger constitutions are like hardwood; they can handle more wear and tear and more stress. Those who are weaker, like softwood, show every bump and scratch. They need more rest and sleep and can't push themselves too far or hard.

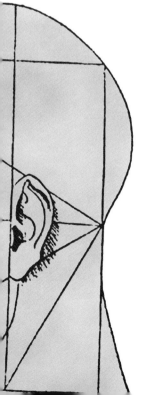

A stronger or yang constitution can be seen in having stronger and bigger bones.

A large head to body ratio is yang; 1:7 is balanced, 1:6 more yang, 1:8 more yin. So taller people tend to be more yin and shorter more yang.

A longer face is more yin and a squarer face is more yang.

Ears reflect the kidneys, which are associated with inherited energy. If they are larger, thicker, lower set, flatter against the head, and larger lobed, then they are more yang.

Body Part Association

Each organ is associated with, or considered to rule, a certain body part and sense organ. **Kidneys rule the bones and joints**, especially the knees and ankles, and may contribute to arthritis because they flush out calcium and other minerals in the urine.

Kidneys have to do with the spine, particularly the lower back.

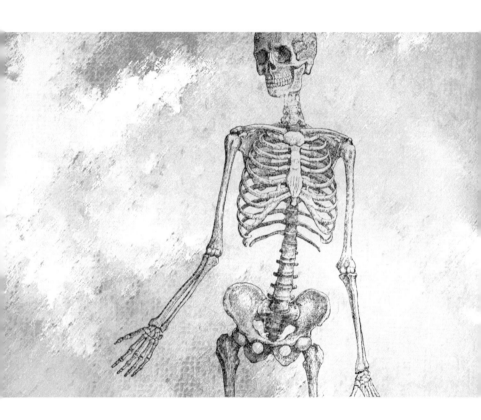

If you break bones easily, then you likely have weak kidneys. Osteoporosis and osteopenia are related to weak kidneys, like you are urinating out your minerals instead of keeping them in place. Depositing minerals in the wrong places, as in kidney stones or in joints contributing to arthritis, is a kidney issue. Low back pain is often due to weak kidneys.

Sense Organ Association

The kidneys correspond to the ears.

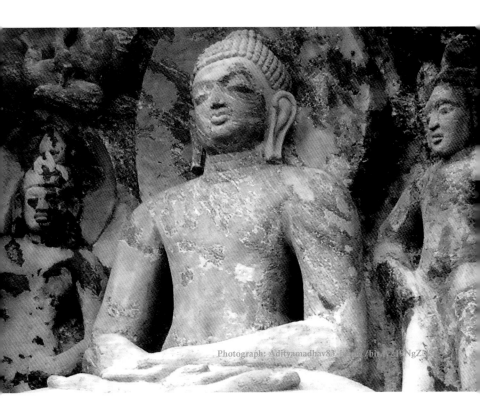

Photograph: Adityamadhav83. /bit.ly/1PNgZR

It is interesting how our ears are shaped like kidneys. There is a map, actually three maps, on the ear that let you treat and diagnose the entire body, as in reflexology. One kidney point is right where the earring hole typically is. A big ear and earlobe is a sign of strong kidneys and thus a long life; look at the earlobes on a Buddha statue! Very old people often have large earlobes. Hearing loss or ringing in the ears is a sign of weak kidneys.

The Taste of Water

The flavor associated with the kidneys and bladder is salty.

Salt is not necessarily good for the kidneys, but it is involved with the kidneys. The World Health Organization advised having one-fifth the salt found in the standard American diet.

Good salt choices: Himalayan or Celtic sea salt, soy sauce, miso (best used in cooking, not raw on food), and gomashio, a sesame salt combination. The sesame oil coats the salt, so it gets into cells.

To grains and vegetables, add a pinch of salt to bring out sweetness. If food tastes salty, you added too much.

Sea salt has 10% magnesium, which calms stress. Table salt has none.

Sea vegetables are high in trace minerals. Have them in a side dish of one to three tsp a day.

Salt should be greatly reduced for those with damp, overweight, lethargic, or edema conditions and for those with high blood pressure.

Salt has a cooling effect and moves energy downward and inward. It softens hardened lumps and stiffness and improves digestion, detoxifies the body, and can purge the bowels.

If you eat salt by itself, you'll crave water or sweet.

Salt can be used in heat conditions such as gargling for a sore throat, brushed with for bleeding gums, or used in a neti pot for inflamed sinuses. It increases appetite and is thus misused in the form of common table salt, which is of poor quality.

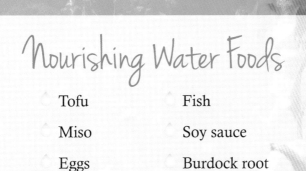

Nourishing Water Foods

Tofu   Fish

Miso   Soy sauce

Eggs   Burdock root

Seaweed vegetables (wakame, kombu, arame, hiziki, kelp, nori, and dulce)

Even though many people should cut back on salt, seaweed is fine to eat. Its iodine and trace minerals actually speed up metabolism.

Much of our soil has been depleted of trace minerals. Seaweeds have all these minerals and a secret missing ingredient in the health of the kidneys. It is said that nori, the wrapper for sushi, is especially good for a weak bladder. Miso soup is an excellent kidney tonic.

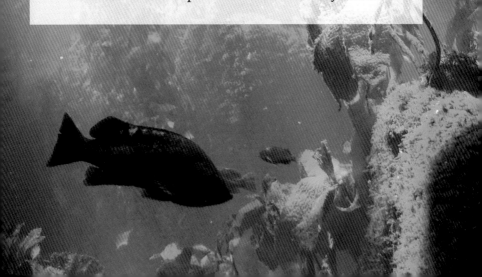

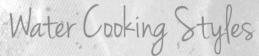

Water Cooking Styles

Water cooking styles include stewing, frying, and nabe (a covered shallow ceramic Japanese pot).

Water is associated with winter. So as salads are great for spring and summer, in the winter, to keep warm and nourish our kidneys we need more stews, which are, of course, watery and you can have more salt than in the warmer seasons.

Frying in oil gives us more calories and fat so we can keep warm in the winter. It is harder for the body to lose weight in the winter because it is in a food-storage mode.

Kidneys/Bladder and Salt

Even though most people abuse low-quality salt and suffer for it, good-quality salt is essential for the health of every cell.

Avoid commercial salt. Instead get sea salt, Celtic sea salt is very healthy, as is Himalayan salt. Both have many trace minerals.

Other good sources of salt are miso, tamari, soy sauce, umeboshi plums (pictured), and sea vegetables.

Salt is very yang and contracting. If eaten in excess it can cause tightness in the body and make one feel too tense.

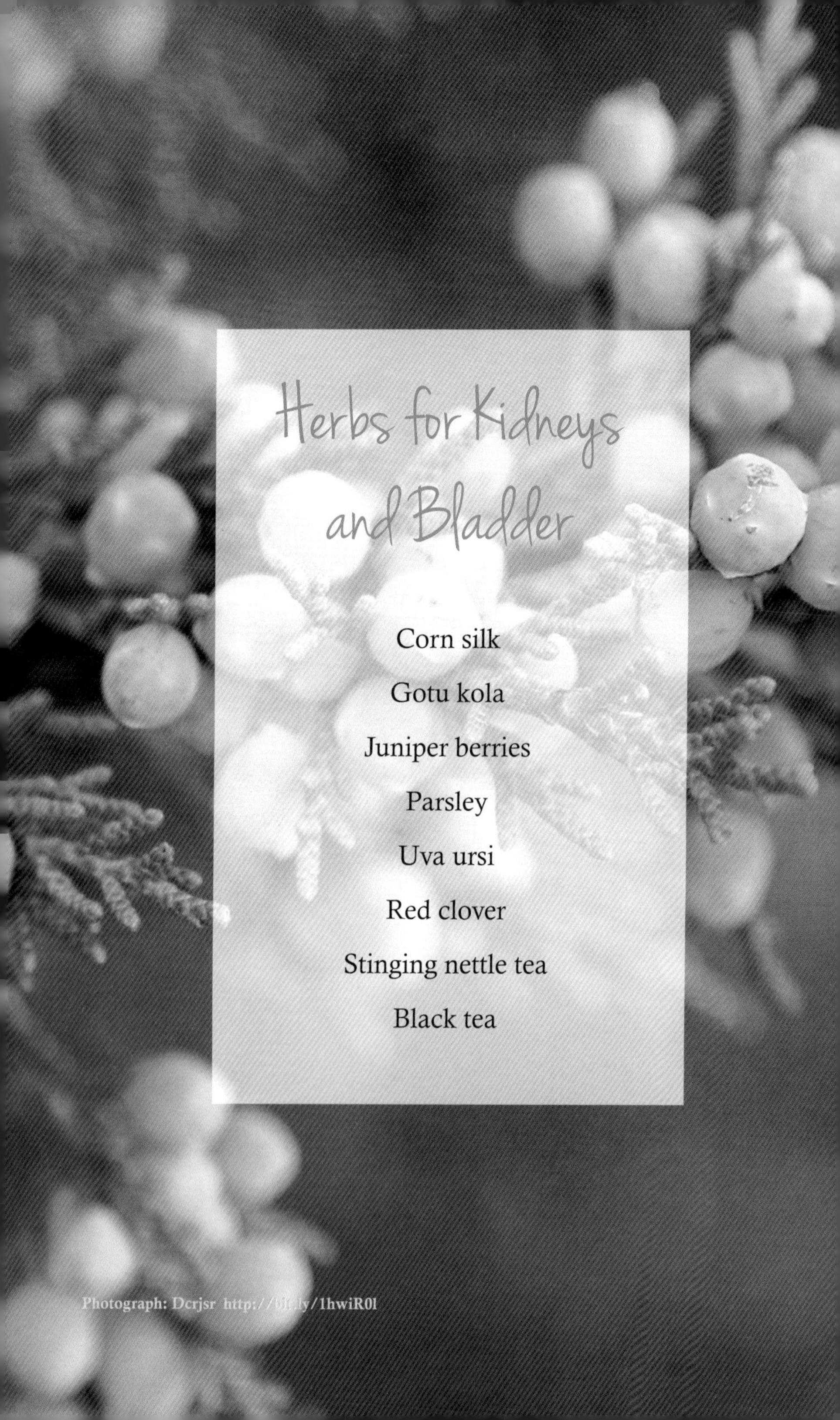

Herbs for Kidneys and Bladder

Corn silk

Gotu kola

Juniper berries

Parsley

Uva ursi

Red clover

Stinging nettle tea

Black tea

Photograph: Dcrjsr http://bit.ly/1hwiR0l

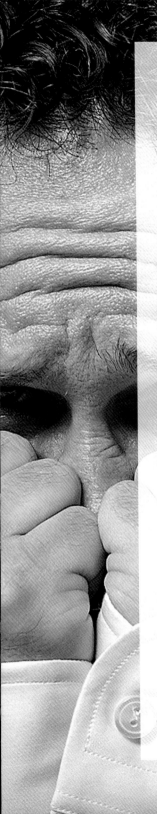

The Kidneys and Emotions

The kidneys are associated with will, memory, and confidence.

Imbalanced kidney energy produces a lack of will, action, and direction.

Fear and anxiety indicate weak kidneys.

If the kidneys are out of balance, you can feel afraid, overwhelmed, confused, and lack confidence. **When in balance, you feel courageous, you know your own mind and feel self-confident and are committed and action oriented.**

Kidney energy has to do with our drive or will in life, including our degree of aggression, sex drive, courage, follow-through, endurance, and right timing.

If the kidneys are too tight and contracted, one can be overly aggressive or violent, stubborn, moving too fast, or insensitive to the space and rhythm of others, often with attachment to the past.

If too tired and swollen, one can be passive, lazy, fearful, lose concern for time, procrastinate or arrive late, lack courage and ambition, and lose appetite for sex or life in general.

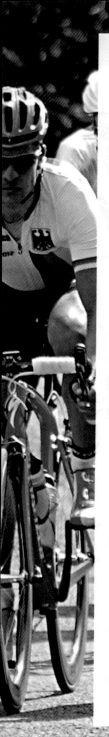

The Spirit of the Kidneys

The spirit that incarnates in the kidneys is called the Zhi.

Psychologically Zhi has to do with instinctual power and is aligned with will and courage.

Forgetfulness, lack of motivation, addiction, depression, fear, sexual issues, sleep disturbance, and controlling others can be signs of an imbalanced Zhi.

Affecting the Zhi

Anytime the will is employed to push the body beyond its own limits; overwork, excessive physical activity, such as excess marathon running, biking, weightlifting.

Use of substances that impinge on adrenal function, such as caffeine, amphetamines, steroids, or cortisone, and chronic disease.

Addictive behavior of any kind, including excess sexual activity, chronic fear and anxiety, particularly during childhood, shock, trauma, and guilt.

Multiple births and excess blood loss during periods.

A lack of discipline and encouragement during childhood.

Photograph: Matt Billings http://bit.ly/1gDYjzM

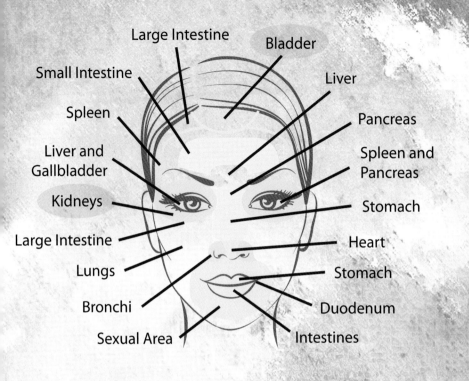

Large Intestine
Bladder
Small Intestine
Liver
Spleen
Pancreas
Liver and Gallbladder
Spleen and Pancreas
Kidneys
Stomach
Large Intestine
Heart
Lungs
Stomach
Bronchi
Duodenum
Sexual Area
Intestines

Facial Diagnosis

The face never lies.

The area below the eyes tells the state of the kidneys.

The chin can also reflect the kidneys and bladder.

Dark or black under the eyes denotes toxic blood due to inadequate detoxification by the kidneys. If skin is drawn and tight under eyes it's a contracted condition. If puffy and swollen it's expanded kidneys. Interestingly, we think of people with a large chin to have more will and a receding chin as being weak willed. This has to do with the inherited kidney energy, which also rules sexuality. A cleft chin is even more contracted or yang, indicating more power.

71

The Kidney Meridian

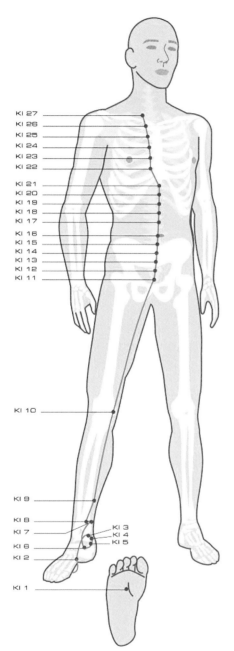

KI 27
KI 26
KI 25
KI 24
KI 23
KI 22
KI 21
KI 20
KI 19
KI 18
KI 17
KI 16
KI 15
KI 14
KI 13
KI 12
KI 11
KI 10
KI 9
KI 8
KI 7
KI 6
KI 2
KI 3
KI 4
KI 5
KI 1

From bottom of foot, around ankle, up inner leg to below the clavicle.

27 acupuncture points.

The kidney is responsible for fluid metabolism and the storage of Jing (essence).

The kidney affects reproduction, teeth, bones, water metabolism, hair loss, and sexual energy.

Meridian can affect lungs, ears, breast, solar plexus, digestion, bladder, and reproductive organs.

Pain, weakness, or skin issues along the meridian, and pain behind the knee and lumbar vertebrae, sacrum and coccyx, as well as pain or skin issues or fungus on soles of feet.

The Bladder Meridian

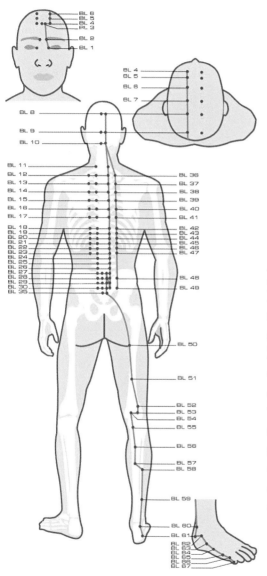

From inside of the eyes, over scalp, along two lines on the sides of the spine, down back of leg to outside of pinky toe.

67 acupuncture points.

The bladder has to do with the excretion of urine.

Meridian issues can be hair loss, headaches, sinus, eye problems, spine pain or stiffness, low back pain, sciatica, calf pain, and weak ankles or feet. Pinky toe is the end of the channel. Research has shown that heating the end point on the outer corner of the pinky nail can turn a breech baby.

Kidney Acupoint

Kidney 3-Taixi-Great Mountain Stream

Location: Midway between inner ankle bone and the Achilles tendon.

Benefits: Fatigue, menstrual irregularities, impotence, low back pain, headache, sore throat, toothache, hearing loss, ringing in the ears, insomnia, swollen feet, ankle pain.

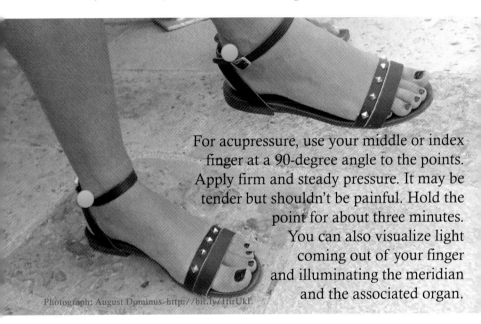

For acupressure, use your middle or index finger at a 90-degree angle to the points. Apply firm and steady pressure. It may be tender but shouldn't be painful. Hold the point for about three minutes. You can also visualize light coming out of your finger and illuminating the meridian and the associated organ.

Photograph: August Dominus-http://bit.ly/1IrUkL

Bladder Acupoint

Bladder 60-Kun Lun-Kunlun Mountain

Location: Midway between the outer ankle bone and the Achilles tendon.

Benefits: Main point for any spine pain, low back pain, pain or numbness in lower limbs, good for excess type headaches where there is too much energy that is stagnant.

Time of Day Water Meridians Peak

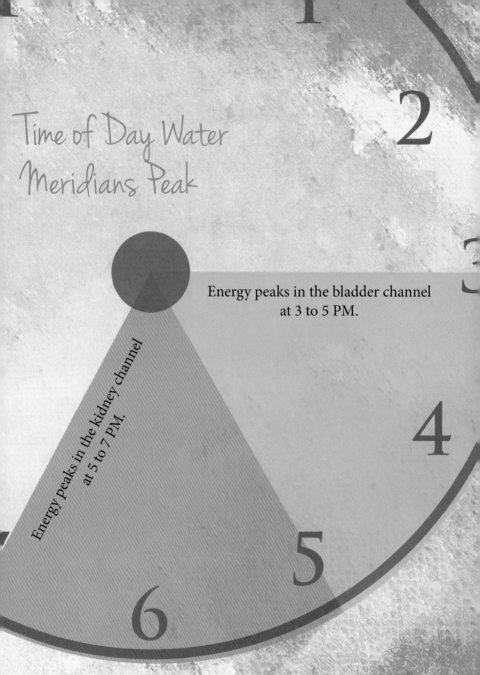

Energy peaks in the bladder channel at 3 to 5 PM.

Energy peaks in the kidney channel at 5 to 7 PM.

If you have an energy drop in the late afternoon, it could indicate a blockage of these organs and meridians. Sometimes you may notice that if you exercise at this time, you have another burst of energy and you won't feel like napping.

Healing Sound for the Kidneys

Qigong has a healing sound for the major organs.
Chui (*chew-eee*) is the sound for the kidneys.

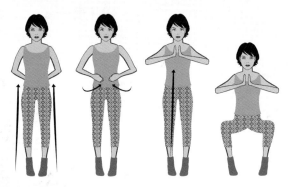

STEP 1: Stand (or sit) with your feet shoulder width apart, arms to your sides. Inhale and raise your hands up toward your lower back with the back of your hands facing your body. As your hands reach kidney level, bring both hands forward toward your belly button with fingers pointing down. As you raise your hands, lead energy up from the bottom of your right foot along the inside of your right leg into the tailbone and along the lower part of your spine into your kidneys. Continue the arm movements and bring your arms in front of your chest until they are right below your collarbone, then turn your palms to face each other. Exhale. Make the *Chui* (*chew-eee*) sound by opening your mouth slightly with your tongue drawn in and the corner of your mouth pulled slightly to the sides. At the same time, squeeze in with your hands as though you were holding a ball, then squat down.

STEP 2: Keep your upper body as straight as you can. Hold up the center of the perineum and pull your abdomen in. As you exhale and make the *Chui* sound, imagine leading all impurities from your kidneys out of your mouth.

STEP 3: Stand up slowly and repeat steps 1 to 2, six times.

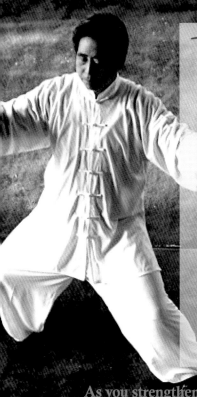

Taking Care of Water

- Nourishing food, rest, meditation, and natural beauty.

- Calming physical exercise, such as yoga, tai chi and qigong.

- Avoidance of excess thinking, working, and craving; maintaining a reasonable schedule and making special time each day to do nothing.

- Spend time with water, get a foot massage, use guided imagery and practice meditation.

As you strengthen your kidneys you will feel empowered instead of drained by life.

Other changes may include the following.

- A sense of power and equilibrium.

- Increased serenity as you stop trying to control the world around you.

- An increased sense of trust.

- The ability to know and speak your authentic feelings and to stay with projects until they are complete.

- Less fear and anxiety, more excitement and curiosity, courage to face the unknown.

- Developing a definite sense of what matters to you, increased initiative, motivation, and perseverance.

- You will be regarded by others as someone to trust.

The Wood Element
Liver and Gallbladder

Wood

The essence of a sprouting grain
Call me wood or tree, it's just a name
An upward rising energy
You may call me ascending chi
Grass, flowers or the mighty oak
I'm the power behind all growth
Though I'm the essence of all humor
When blocked I can even grow a tumor
Present at spring, I give rebirth
Behind all laughter, I am mirth
Upward and onward, my motto and song
I see what's right and not what's wrong
I wake each bird and every child
I'm in the wind that runneth wild
The mist that rises in the morn
Each new day is the sun reborn
For all those yearning to be free
Look within and look to me.

—Warren King

Energy of Wood

Don't think of wood energy as a piece of wood.

Think of it more as a living tree.

Energy is moving upward, like sap moves up a tree.

Or water evaporating into clouds.

If you have a hard time waking up in the morning, it is likely that the gentle upward energy of wood is not free flowing.

"The Light Fall" ©2018 Connie Kroskin

Wood in the Daily Cycle

🌱 Since wood is upward energy,
it has to do with the sunrise.

🌱 Wood rules the energy of the morning.

🌱 Think of birds singing in the morning.

🌱 Is it hard to wake up?

Wood in the Yearly Cycle

🌱 Spring is like the sunrise of the year.

🌱 Everything is moving upward.

🌱 If you feel worse in the spring, such as having
allergies, you could have a wood imbalance.

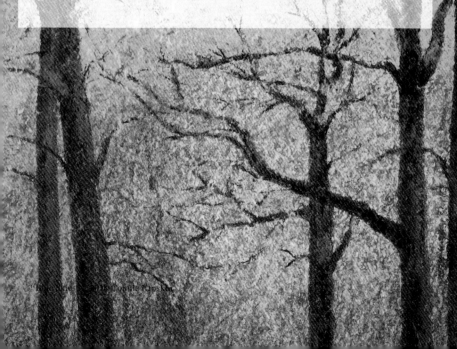

The liver is the largest and most complex organ of the body.

🌳 The liver affects nearly every physiological process of the body and performs over 500 different chemical functions.

🌳 One-third of all blood in the body passes through the liver every minute, about 1.5 quarts. It detoxifies the blood by filtering out toxins that assault your body on a regular basis.

🌳 It also helps with hormonal balance, fat regulation, and digestion.

🌳 Carbohydrates, fats, and proteins can all be changed into one another by the liver. Excess food that is not used can be turned into fat or mucus.

🌳 If 80% of the liver is destroyed by sickness or surgery, it can grow back quickly, all the while carrying on its normal functions.

🌳 The liver stores certain vitamins, minerals, and sugars and produces quick energy when it is needed.

🌳 It controls the production and excretion of cholesterol and produces immune factors that help the body fight off infection.

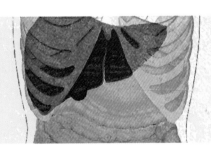

You should be able to get your fingers underneath your right rib cage. If it's like cement you may have compacted fat in the liver.

Wood Element Organs

Wood corresponds to the liver.

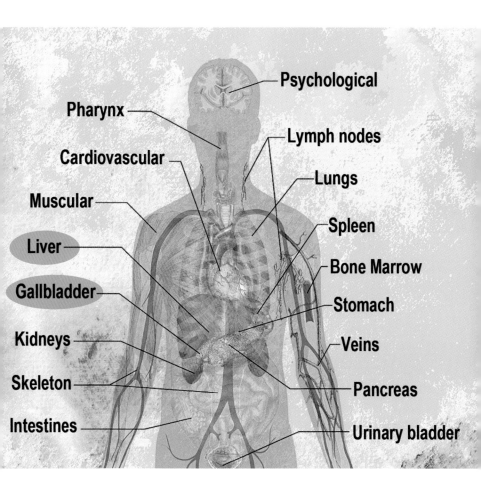

When the liver is out of balance, there is a blockage of energy and in the flow of fluids. Tendons are not moistened and can easily tear, become inflamed, or cause unusual contraction or weakness in their related muscles. A common result of liver stagnation is an inflexible and rigid body.

Paired Organ of Wood

The hollow organ that is paired with
the liver is the gallbladder.

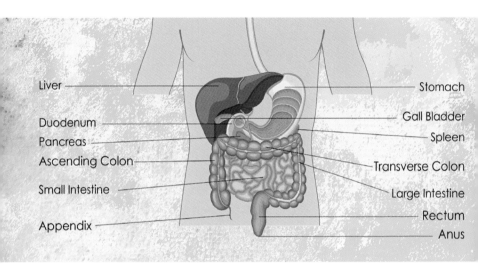

Liver — Stomach

Duodenum — Gall Bladder

Pancreas — Spleen

Ascending Colon — Transverse Colon

Small Intestine — Large Intestine

Rectum

Appendix — Anus

The gallbladder stores about two ounces of bile, which is released when food containing fat enters the digestive tract. The bile emulsifies fats and neutralizes acids in partly digested food. Bile is made of three parts. One is bile salt made from cholesterol, one is a pigment from dead red blood cells that give stool a brownish color, and another is waste and toxins.

The condition of the gallbladder is dependent on our intake of fats and oils. Americans eat 300 pounds of dairy products and 200 pounds of meat a year, plus 35 pounds of oils. These fats can solidify in the gallbladder and create stones.

If the gallbladder has been removed, it can't store bile and the liver must work harder from then on. You can live fine but need to limit fat and consume more sour foods.

Cold drinks can solidify fats in the gallbladder. We drink about 1.5 quarts of 40-degree liquids a day.

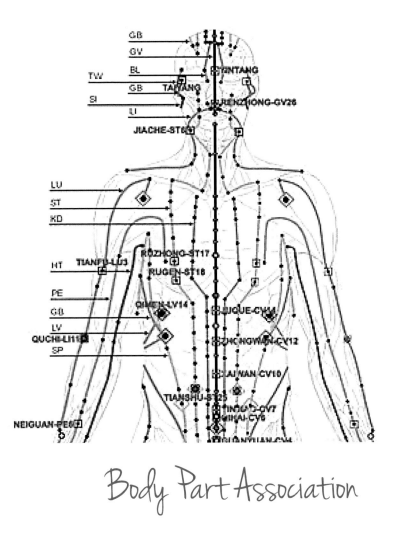

Body Part Association

Each organ is associated with, or considered to rule, a certain body part and sense organ.

Liver rules the ligaments and tendons.
It has a relation to the shoulders.

The liver meridian passes through the eyes. Cataracts, glaucoma, red or dry eyes, night blindness, excessive tearing, far- and nearsightedness, and other eye conditions reflect the condition of the liver.

Sense Organ Association

The liver corresponds to the eyes.

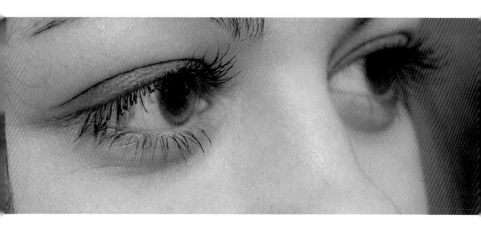

🌿 If the whites of the eyes look yellowish or get crusty (or regular visits from the sandman) in the morning, the cause is fat accumulation in the liver.

🌿 If eyes are red or bloodshot or if you get red spots or styes on the eyes, lids, or between the eyes, it's due to a swollen and inflamed liver.

🌿 If eyes are watery or swollen or burn or itch, it's from a swollen liver. Dryness is an overly contracted condition.

I have seen many eye conditions cleared up merely by addressing the liver and not even treating the eyes directly.

I have found that sudden bloody spots on the whites of the eyes often happen after eating a combination of too much fat with sweet, like ice cream or chocolate.

The Taste of Wood

The flavor associated with the liver
and gallbladder is sour.

Sour flavor has a
dispersing effect on the liver, so
this is good if the liver is tight and full of
fat. To help the liver deal with fat and oil add
more green vegetables like broccoli, collards, and
scallions.

If you wake up grouchy, it's due to liver stagnation. When
wood energy is flowing smoothly you have patience. If you're
tense and irritable and angry at traffic, you may need to eat less
oil and saturated fat.

Fermented vegetables are a good source for the sour flavor.
Vegetable juices can also reduce excess in the liver, especially with
greens. So add celery, kale, or parsley to your carrot juice.

The sour flavor can help with abnormal leakage of
fluid or energy such as urinary dripping, excess
perspiration, hemorrhage, and diarrhea. It
can also firm up tissues in cases such as
flaccid skin, hemorrhoids, and
uterine prolapse.

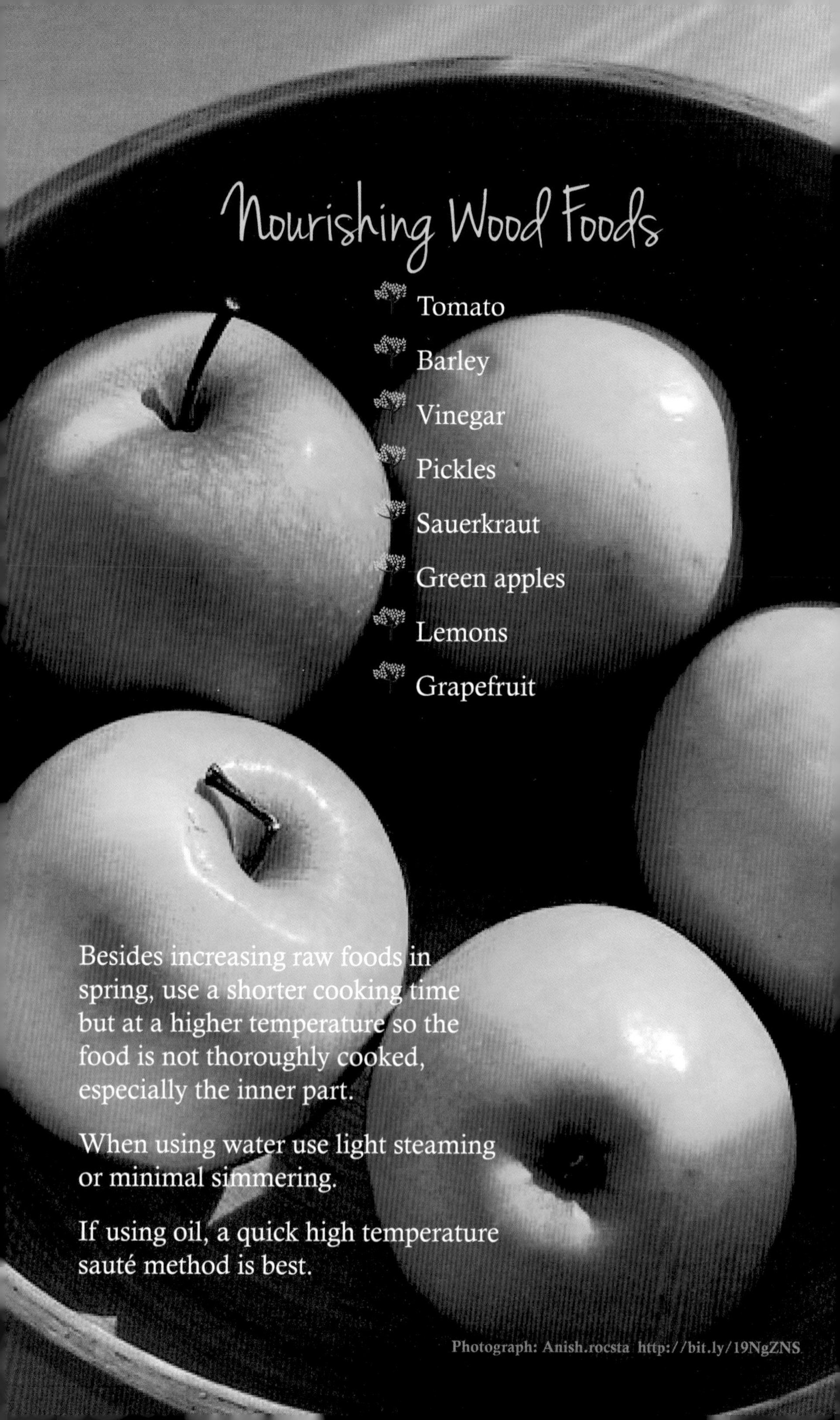

Nourishing Wood Foods

- Tomato
- Barley
- Vinegar
- Pickles
- Sauerkraut
- Green apples
- Lemons
- Grapefruit

Besides increasing raw foods in spring, use a shorter cooking time but at a higher temperature so the food is not thoroughly cooked, especially the inner part.

When using water use light steaming or minimal simmering.

If using oil, a quick high temperature sauté method is best.

Photograph: Anish.rocsta http://bit.ly/19NgZNS

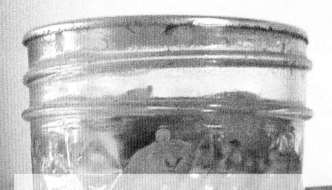

Wood Cooking Styles

Wood cooking styles include: pickling, blanching, pressed salad, or steaming. Grilling, smoking, and steaming are also associated with the wood element.

For a pressed salad, massage shredded vegetables with salt, then put them in a pickle press or put a plate over the veggies with a weight on top until water comes out of the vegetables. You can try this with lettuce, radishes, cucumbers, or spinach, and press for about 24 hours.

Liver/Gallbladder and Oils

Bile made in the liver is stored in the gallbladder, which secretes it into the small intestine to emulsify and digest oils.

Avoid low-quality oils such as cottonseed, canola, corn, and soy. The best oils are olive, coconut, sesame, and grapeseed.

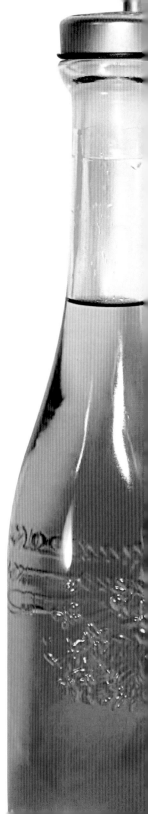

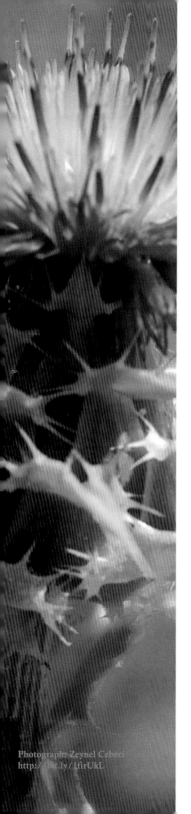

Herbs for Liver

❦ **Dandelion** is an overall liver cleanser and tonic. It is particularly effective for premenstrual mood swings accompanied by bloating and breast tenderness.

❦ **Peppermint** is a mood-elevating, invigorating herb that also helps with digestive disturbances, bloating, and poor appetite. Take as a tea and drink freely throughout the day.

❦ **Burdock root** cleanses the liver and blood, can be cooked when fresh, like a carrot, or used in a tea when dried.

❦ **Milk thistle** is the premier herb for anyone who has been exposed to toxic chemicals. It should be taken for at least two months after exposure. It is beneficial for people who work with chemicals or are routinely exposed to pollution.

❦ **Chelidonium** is one of the best overall liver tonics. It should be taken as a tincture—a few drops in a tablespoon of water—three times a day before meals, and it will quickly clear digestive and appetite disturbances, enhance clarity of vision, and ease emotional strain.

The Liver and Emotions

Planning ability and good judgment are marks of a healthy liver.

Emotions related to anger are one of the first signs of a liver imbalance: impatience, frustration, resentment, violence, belligerence, rudeness, arrogance, stubbornness, aggression, and an impulsive or explosive personality. If these are repressed, they can cause depression.

The gallbladder is small, so little angers like frustration and irritability can show up. Mood swings and emotional excesses in general are liver related.

A healthy liver ensures patience, alertness, endurance, perseverance, the energetic pursuit of spiritual development, and the maintenance of a strong spiritual center.

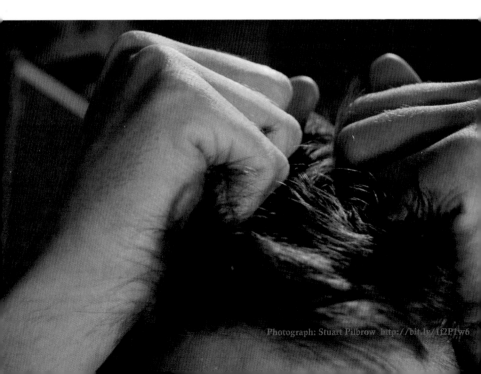

The Spirit of Liver

The spirit that incarnates in the liver is called the Hun. It has to do with vision, imagination, dreams, direction, decision, and justice. It also has to do with benevolence and finding one's true path.

As you work with and heal your liver, the home for the Hun, you should achieve…

- More clarity and direction in your life purpose.

- Increased ability to achieve your goals with less procrastination.

- Better imagination and guidance through day and night dreams.

- More emotional stability with the ability to know what you're feeling and stand by your feelings and beliefs.

- Less indecisiveness, guilt, timidity, irritability, and depression.

- More passion and excitement in life with zest and a more colorful life.

- Less blaming of others and feeling that life is unfair.

"Crossing Path" ©2018 Connie Kroskin

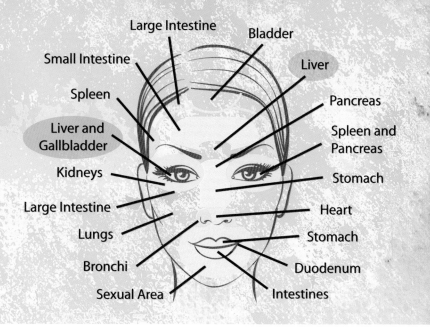

Large Intestine

Bladder

Small Intestine

Liver

Spleen

Pancreas

Liver and
Gallbladder

Spleen and
Pancreas

Kidneys

Stomach

Large Intestine

Heart

Lungs

Stomach

Bronchi

Duodenum

Sexual Area

Intestines

Facial Diagnosis

Ⴤ **The face never lies.**

Ⴤ The area between the eyebrows indicates the state of the liver.

Ⴤ The gallbladder is outside that area and near the hairline at the edges of forehead.

In general, redness or puffiness is related to yin or expansive energy. This can be from sugar or excess sweets, citrus, chemicals, spices, vinegar, or alcohol. Tightness or darker colors can be from too much yang or contractive energy, perhaps from too much meat, eggs, cheese, or salt. White colorations can be from many milk products.

A deep line between the eyebrows means the liver is overly contracted. If there are several shallow vertical lines the liver is overly expanded.

Remember that the color of the wood element is green, so a greenish complexion or patches can relate to liver or gallbladder, but also can be a precancerous sign.

The Liver Meridian

꙳ From the inside of the big toe, up inner leg to groin to under breast.

꙳ 14 acupuncture points.

꙳ The liver stores the blood and is responsible for maintaining the free flow of Qi throughout the body.

꙳ The liver can affect digestion, menstruation, tendons and ligaments, bile production, and eye problems.

Some problems related to the liver meridian: uterus or prostate problems, genital problems, inner knee and thigh pain, skin issues or varicose veins, big toe problems like gout or nail fungus, or ingrown toenail.

Besides traversing just below the surface of the skin, meridians also dive deeper into the body in an internal pathway.

In addition to the meridian flow along the skin, there are deeper internal pathways. Problems with the internal pathways can cause diaphragm and lung conditions, tightness in the chest, the feeling of something in the throat (plum pit) and eye pain.

LR 14
LR 13
LR 12
LR 11
LR 10
LR 9
LR 8
LR 7
LR 6
LR 5
LR 4
LR 3
LR 2
LR 1

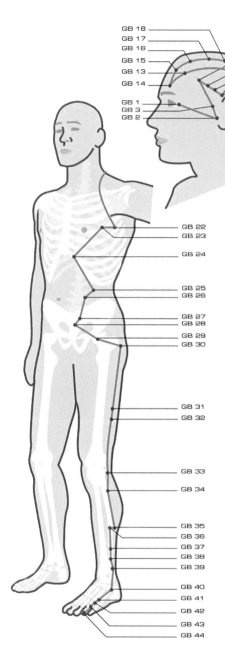

GB 18
GB 17
GB 16
GB 15
GB 13
GB 14
GB 1
GB 3
GB 2

GB 4
GB 5
GB 6
GB 8
GB 9
GB 7
GB 10
GB 19
GB 11
GB 12
GB 20

GB 21

GB 22
GB 23
GB 24
GB 25
GB 26
GB 27
GB 28
GB 29
GB 30
GB 31
GB 32
GB 33
GB 34
GB 35
GB 36
GB 37
GB 38
GB 39
GB 40
GB 41
GB 42
GB 43
GB 44

The Gallbladder Meridian

From the outside of the eyes, the side of the head, the side of the chest, to outside of the leg, to the outside of the fourth toe.

The gallbladder governs the storage and secretion of bile that is received by the liver.

Symptoms of imbalance with this meridian can be pain in face, head, jaw, neck, or occiput. Pain and stiffness can occur in the shoulders, ribs, hips, and outer legs. There can be skin issues, such as shingles, and problems with the fourth toe or toenail. Problems with the fourth toe or toenail.

Liver Acupoint

Liver 3-Taichong-Supreme Rushing

Location: Slide your finger up between the second and big toe on top of the foot, in the valley where the bones come together.

Benefits: Helps the liver, good for migraines, menstrual problems, digestive disorders, irritability, insomnia, dizziness, exhaustion, and headaches.

For stress, tension, and to clear the head, treat this point along with Large Intestine 4 (see page 51), called the Four Gates.

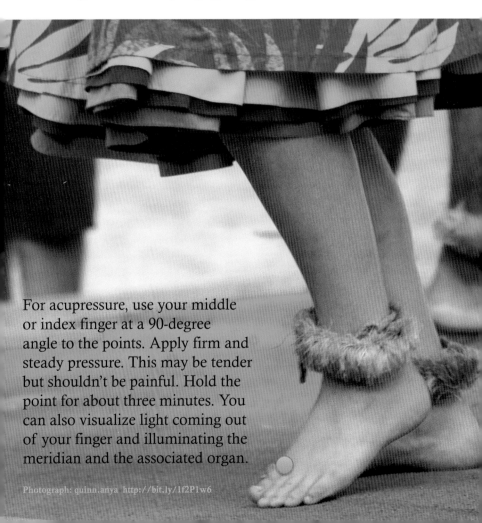

For acupressure, use your middle or index finger at a 90-degree angle to the points. Apply firm and steady pressure. This may be tender but shouldn't be painful. Hold the point for about three minutes. You can also visualize light coming out of your finger and illuminating the meridian and the associated organ.

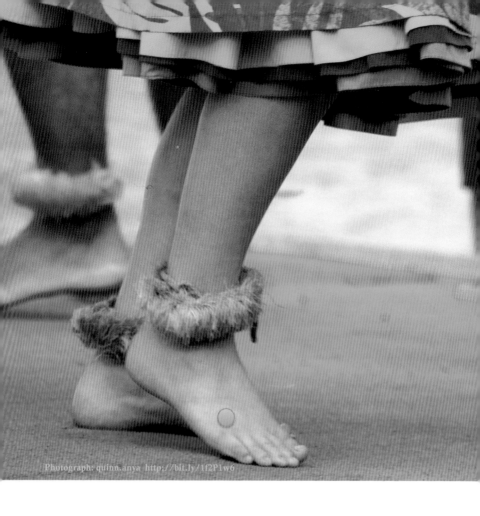

Gallbladder Acupoint

Gallbladder 41-Zulingqi-Foot Near to Tears

Location: On the top side of the foot, slide up one inch between the fourth and fifth toes, in the groove between the bones.

Benefits: Hip pain, shoulder tension, moving joint pains, headaches, dizziness, side aches, water retention, sciatic, and foot pain.

Time of Day Wood Meridians Peak

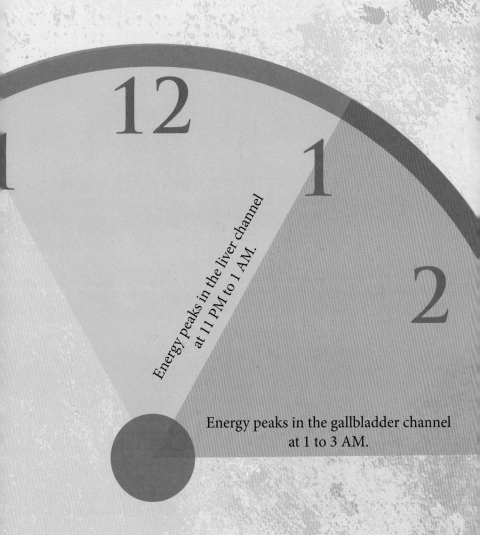

Energy peaks in the liver channel at 11 PM to 1 AM.

Energy peaks in the gallbladder channel at 1 to 3 AM.

Healing Sound for the Liver

Qigong has a healing sound for the major organs.

Xu (pronounced *shu-yii*)

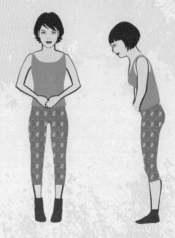

STEP 1: Stand naturally. Overlap your hands on top of your abdomen. Men: place your left hand a few finger spaces below the navel. Women: place your right hand on the same area.

STEP 2: Inhale. Imagine leading energy from your right big toe up the inside of your right leg past the reproductive organs, up below your right rib cage and up just below your right breast.

STEP 3: Exhale. Open your eyes wide and mentally look into your liver. Let out the *Xu* (*shu-yii*) sound as you lean forward slightly. At the same time, hold up the center of your perineum and draw your abdomen in to squeeze out the impurities from your liver. Repeat for six inhalations and exhalations.

The Fire Element
Heart and
Small Intestine

Fire

I am the fire of the Central Sun
The light of life, of everyone
The heat that keeps the bloodstream warm
The lightning of the thunderstorm
Wisdom of the sage's mind
All impure I shall refine
Bees buzzing on a summer day
Children jumping, as they laugh and play
Quasars, pulsars, electrons, too
All that's old I shall renew
The hearth that comforts every home
I breathe in every centrosome
The glint in every warrior's eye
The faith that martyrs never die
The glow of cosmos, the light of space
The speed of thought, desire to race
Beyond all form and every name
Behold, I beat thine own heart flame.

—Warren King

Energy of Fire

Fire is the most expansive energy.

It is upward and outward.

Flames are always moving upward.

It is a more extreme energy that occurs between wood energy, which is gently moving upward, and earth energy, which is beginning to settle.

Fire in the Daily Cycle

🔥 Since fire is the most upward energy, it has to do with the time when the sun is highest in the sky.

🔥 So fire energy peaks around noon.

🔥 We are most awake at that time.

Fire in the Yearly Cycle

🔥 Summer is like the noontime of the year.

🔥 Fire moves upward and outward.

🔥 There is a literal buzzing energy in summer; the crickets, cicadas, birds, and frogs are singing.

Most people love summer. Everything is blossoming, nature is noisy and bustling with energy. People often take time off from school and work and play more and spend time outside, although sometimes it can get too hot. We don't want to cook very much in a hot kitchen.

Fire Element Organs

Fire corresponds to the heart.

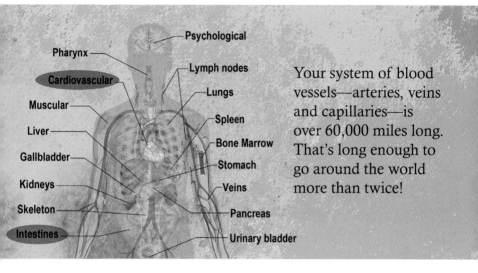

Pharynx
Cardiovascular
Muscular
Liver
Gallbladder
Kidneys
Skeleton
Intestines

Psychological
Lymph nodes
Lungs
Spleen
Bone Marrow
Stomach
Veins
Pancreas
Urinary bladder

Your system of blood vessels—arteries, veins and capillaries—is over 60,000 miles long. That's long enough to go around the world more than twice!

🔥 The adult heart pumps about five quarts of blood each minute, approximately 2,000 gallons of blood each day throughout the body. That's 400 five-gallon bottles.

🔥 The heart beats about 100,000 times each day. In a 70-year lifetime, the average human heart beats more than 2.5 billion times.

🔥 A child's heart is about the size of a clenched fist; an adult's heart is about the size of two fists.

🔥 Blood takes about 20 seconds to circulate throughout the entire vascular system.

🔥 Expansive foods weaken the heart: sugar, alcohol, coffee, caffeine. They are yin and can cause the heart to swell and beat irregularly. A fatty, compacted heart is a more yang condition. If you eat the standard American diet for 30 to 60 years you will get blockages from hard fats, meats, eggs, and cheese.

Paired Organ of Fire

The hollow organ paired with the heart is the small intestine

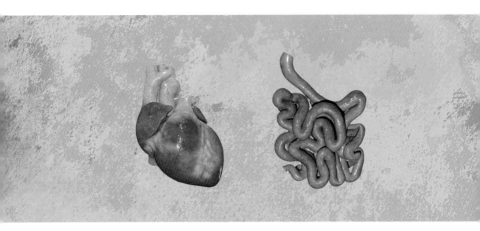

* The small intestine is about 23 feet long and 1.5 inches wide. About 90% of what we eat is assimilated (enters the blood) in the small intestine.

* Food is alkalized in the small intestine with the help of enzymes secreted from the pancreas and gallbladder. It has a huge surface area, 10 times greater than the skin, with folds and villi (finger-like projections) with smaller villi on them.

* Food goes from the small intestine to the liver via the portal vein, but fat goes directly into the lymphatic system. Leaky gut is a very common and serious problem. When the tight junctions between the cells break down and the villi become permeable, then whole molecules of proteins can get into the bloodstream. The body perceives these as being invaders and launches an immune response and you can end up with a food allergy. Worse than that is the fact that these antibodies can then target the body's own cells, which are similar to the foods. So instead of just attacking the wheat gluten molecule, the immune system can attack your own pancreas cells and create diabetes.

Body Part Association

Each organ is associated with, or considered to rule, a certain body part and sense organ. **Heart rules the blood vessels.**

So varicose veins or bruising easily may indicate a problem with the heart energy.

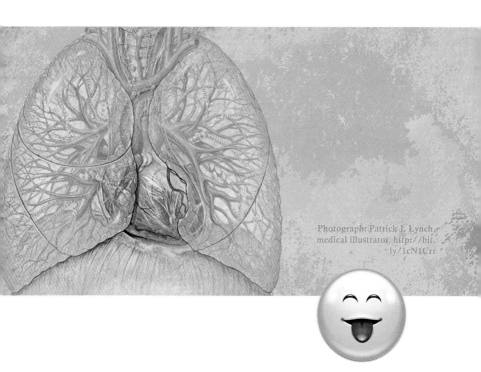

Photograph: Patrick J. Lynch, medical illustrator http://bit. ly/1cN1Crr

Sense Organ Association

The heart corresponds to the tongue (called the sprout of the heart).

A sore on your tongue may indicate heat in the heart meridian. Stuttering or stammering in speech can indicate a heart murmur or hyperactive heartbeat. These can also lead to jerky kinds of movements, or the inability to sit still or get comfortable.

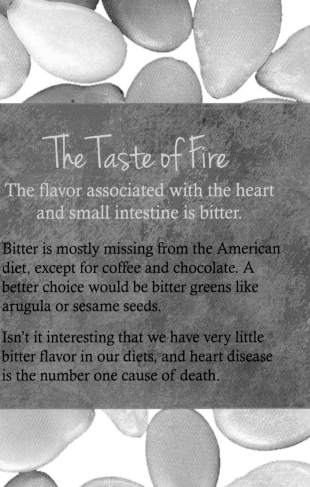

The Taste of Fire

The flavor associated with the heart and small intestine is bitter.

Bitter is mostly missing from the American diet, except for coffee and chocolate. A better choice would be bitter greens like arugula or sesame seeds.

Isn't it interesting that we have very little bitter flavor in our diets, and heart disease is the number one cause of death.

Nourishing Fire Foods

Bitter is eaten in the least quantity of all the five tastes but we should have it regularly.

- Kale
- Dandelion
- Arugula
- Sesame seeds
- Bitter greens
- Daikon radish
- Brussel sprouts
- Celery
- Lettuce
- Broccoli
- Endive
- Collard greens
- Quinoa
- Orange peel
- Kumquats
- Black currants

- **Shiitake mushroom** helps clear cholesterol from blood vessels. Cholesterol sticks more if the blood vessels are damaged by high sugar in the blood.

- The heart likes a rhythmic life: regular sleeping, waking, and eating times.

- A fatty meal makes platelets stick together like sludge for six hours, then another meal is eaten so the blood never flows well. All organs and cells depend on good circulation.

- Bitter helps to lower blood pressure, and **celery** is specifically good for this. Bitter is said to drain dampness, so it is good for Candida yeast overgrowth, parasites, mucus, skin eruptions, tumors, cysts, edema, and obesity.

- Bitter foods are especially good for those who are slow, overweight, lethargic and damp or watery, and also good for overheated and aggressive people. On the other hand, those who are thin, cold, weak, and nervous should limit bitter.

Photograph: Tiia Monto   http://bit.ly/1UAZN8

Fire Cooking Styles

- Food preparations include raw, pressed salad, stir frying, and blanching, as well as toasting and dehydration. Appetizers and snacks are also ruled by the fire element.

- Besides increasing raw foods in spring, when cooking, it should be with a shorter cooking time but at a higher temperature, so the food is not cooked through, especially the inner part.

- When using water, use light steaming or minimal simmering. If you use oil then a quick high temperature sauté method is best.

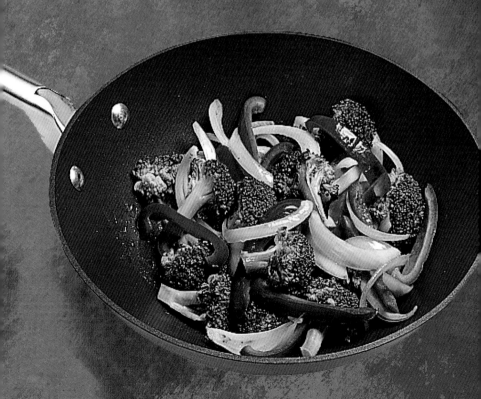

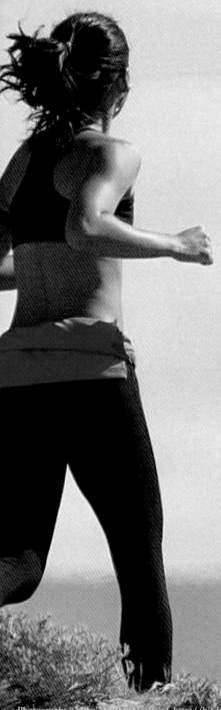

Heart and Exercise

🔥 People with an active lifestyle have 45% less heart disease than sedentary people.

🔥 Sedentary people have a 35% higher incidence of high blood pressure than active people.

🔥 Exercise helps cholesterol levels and reduces inflammation in the arteries.

🔥 It is recommended to get 150 minutes of moderate, or 75 minutes of vigorous exercise a week.

Herbs for Heart

- Hawthorne
- Chickweed
- Garlic
- Olive leaf
- Hawthorn
- Lavender
- Green tea
- Oregano
- Cayenne
- Olive leaf

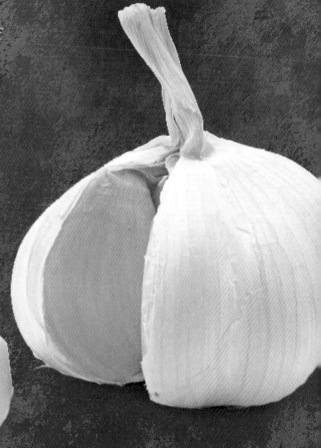

Photograph: Dubravko Soric http://bit.ly/1gDYjzM

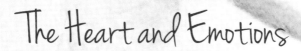

The Heart and Emotions

Joy is the emotion of the heart when balanced.

An imbalanced heart can result in the following.

* Panic or hysteria.

* Some psychological difficulties involving defective self-image.

* Problems with relationships in general.

The heart is like the central headquarters for incoming information from the other organs. With a heart out of balance, a person can be overexcited, too tense, unable to enjoy life, or a workaholic. **When balanced you feel more relaxed, playful, lighter, inspired, and celebratory.**

The Spirit of the Heart

🔥 The spirit that incarnates in the heart is called the Shen.

🔥 It is the fiery spark of consciousness and is reflected in the light shining from the eyes.

🔥 Its virtues are compassion and love.

🔥 Sleeping problems and disturbed dreams are Shen imbalances.

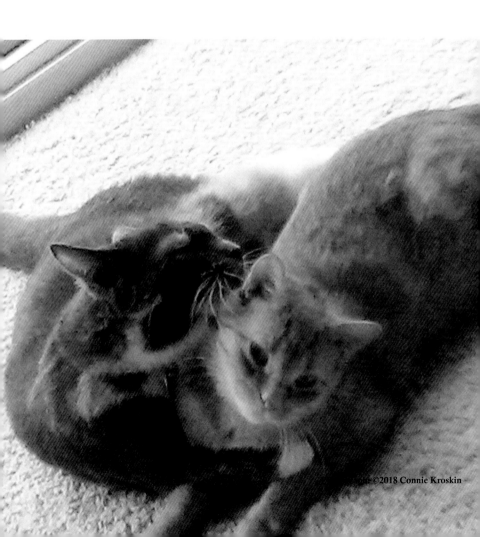

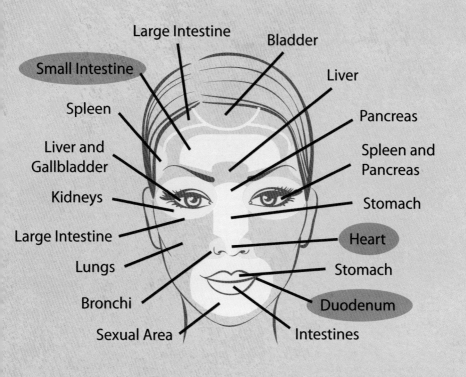

Large Intestine
Bladder
Small Intestine
Liver
Spleen
Pancreas
Liver and Gallbladder
Spleen and Pancreas
Kidneys
Stomach
Large Intestine
Heart
Lungs
Stomach
Bronchi
Duodenum
Sexual Area
Intestines

Facial Diagnosis

🔥 **The face never lies.**

🔥 The nose represents the state of the heart.

🔥 The small intestine can be reflected in the corners of the mouth and inside of the lips as well as the middle of the forehead.

Facial Diagnosis

A swollen or reddish face may mean a heart issue, with redness indicating high blood pressure, especially if there are expanded capillaries of the nose.

Purple on the tip of the nose indicates that the heart is weak and has lost much of its elasticity and strength, and may mean low blood pressure, a more advanced condition than if red.

Waxy pallor on some noses are fat deposits surrounding the heart, usually too much saturated fat in the diet. Herbs like ginger, scallions, garlic, and daikon radish can melt away these fat deposits.

When you have cracks or sores on the corners of the mouth, it usually indicates poor food combinations, as do sores on the inside of your lips. Sometimes we bite our lips when chewing, that is usually due to an inflammation of the inside of the lips, which reflects an inflamed small intestine.

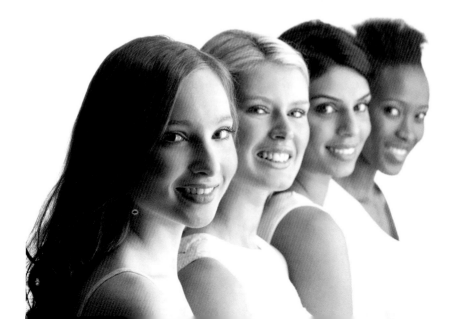

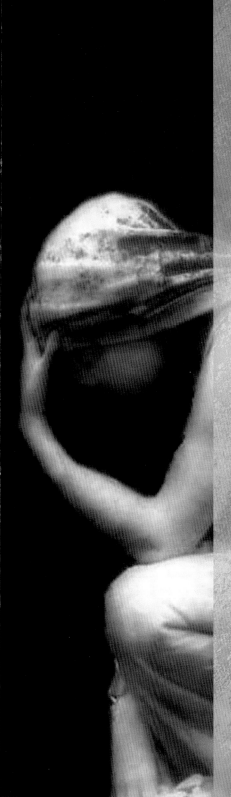

Balance

Shen (Spirit) Imbalances

- Anxiety
- Palpitations
- Difficulty concentrating
- Being timid or easily startled
- Being overly talkative—remember that the heart rules the tongue
- Mania or schizophrenia
- Being incoherent in speech
- Being hyperactive and restless

Person with a Balanced Shen

- Unique individual with a unique path
- Has self-reflection and can distinguish the true from the unreal

Anything that upsets the heart upsets the Shen. Emotional trauma, shock, and abuse can cause a Shen disturbance, as can recreational drugs and excessive alcohol.

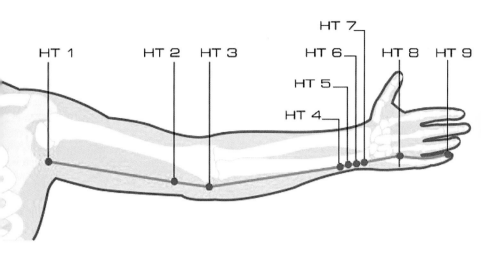

The Heart Meridian

🔥 From underarm to inside of the pinky finger.

🔥 Nine acupuncture points.

🔥 The heart governs the circulation of blood and is the residence of Shen (spirit) and has to do with clear thinking.

🔥 Shen disturbance may manifest as insomnia, excess dreaming, or forgetfulness. A more seriously imbalanced condition may include hysteria, irrational behavior, insanity, or delirium.

Other disorders may include palpitations or skipped beats, rapid heartbeat, chest pain, and heart disorders.

A meridian disorder can give numbness, stiffness, or pain along the inner arm or the pinky finger or nail. Pain or swollen glands in the armpit can be heart related.

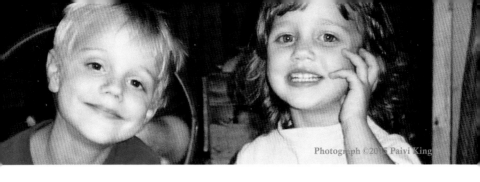

Small Intestine Meridian

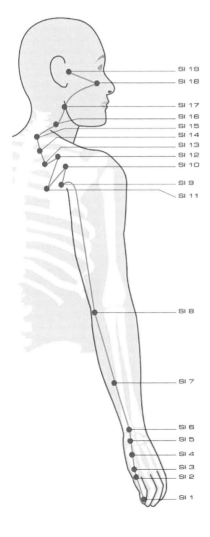

SI 19
SI 18
SI 17
SI 16
SI 15
SI 14
SI 13
SI 12
SI 10
SI 9
SI 11
SI 8
SI 7
SI 6
SI 5
SI 4
SI 3
SI 2
SI 1

🔥 From outside of the pinky finger to scapula to in front of the ear.

🔥 21 acupuncture points.

🔥 Receives food from the stomach.

🔥 Separates nutrition from waste.

The small intestine meridian goes to the ears and face, so hearing loss or facial neuralgia may be signs of imbalance. Also there might be swollen lymph nodes in the throat and scapula or shoulder pain or skin issues along the meridian to the outer pinky.

I used to get pain on my outer pinky nail if I had eaten bad food combinations.

119

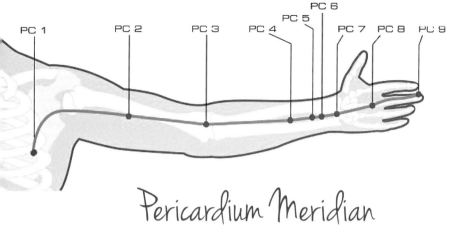

PC 1   PC 2   PC 3   PC 4   PC 5   PC 6   PC 7   PC 8   PC 9

Pericardium Meridian

- The pericardium is called the "heart protector."

- It is also considered a fire element organ.

- If the heart is the "emperor," then the pericardium is the "ambassador."

- It is the first line of defense protecting the heart from external pathogenic influence.

- Often the heart is treated in acupuncture not directly but through the pericardium meridian.

- Nine points, starting near the nipple down inside of the arm to the tip of the middle finger.

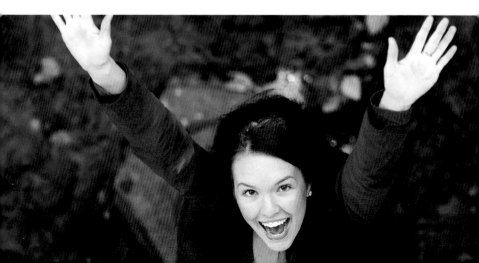

Triple Warmer Meridian

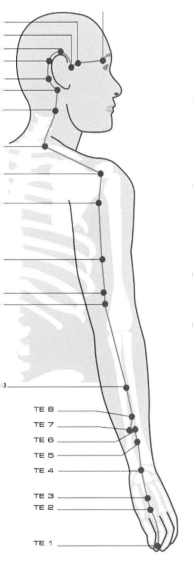

- The only meridian that has no corresponding physical organ.

- It is paired with the pericardium and is also considered part of the fire element.

- It consist of three warmers: upper in chest, middle in stomach area, and lower in lower abdomen.

- It has to do with metabolism and digestion.

- From the ring finger, up the middle of outside of the arm, to the shoulder, to the ear to outside of the eyebrow.

TE 8
TE 7
TE 6
TE 5
TE 4

TE 3
TE 2

TE 1

Heart Acupoint

Heart 7-Shen Men-Spirit Gate

Location: On the inner wrist crease, in line with the pinky, on the thumb side of the tendon.

Benefits: Insomnia from overexcitement, anxiety, heart problems or pain, palpitations, mental or emotional imbalances, irritability, or headache.

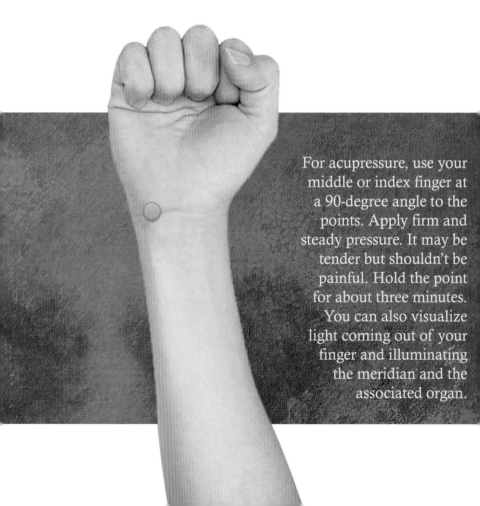

For acupressure, use your middle or index finger at a 90-degree angle to the points. Apply firm and steady pressure. It may be tender but shouldn't be painful. Hold the point for about three minutes. You can also visualize light coming out of your finger and illuminating the meridian and the associated organ.

Small Intestine Acupoint

Small Intestine 3-Hou Xi-Back Ravine

Location: On outside of the hand on the pinky side. When you make a fist, it is the high point on the crease above the pinky.

Benefits: Tinnitus (ringing in the ears), stiff neck, back pain, occipital pain, night sweats, dizziness, earache, sore throat, anxiety, and manic depression.

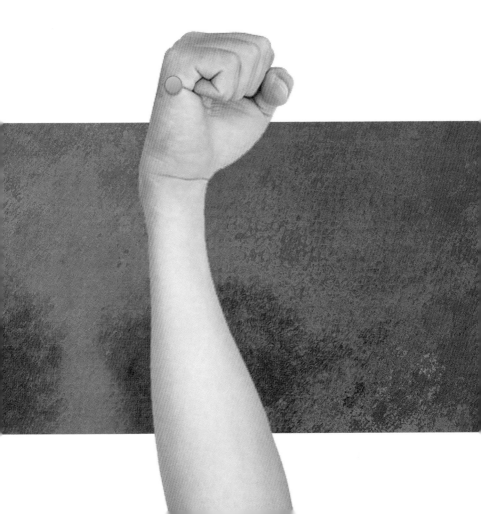

Pericardium Acupoint

Pericardium 6-Nei Guan-Inner Pass

Location: Two thumb widths from the wrist crease on the inner forearm between the two tendons.

Benefits: Nausea, motion sickness, hiccups, vomiting, stomach grumbling, abdominal pain, or distention. Good for tightness in the chest, palpitations, anxiety, shortness of breath, as well as insomnia.

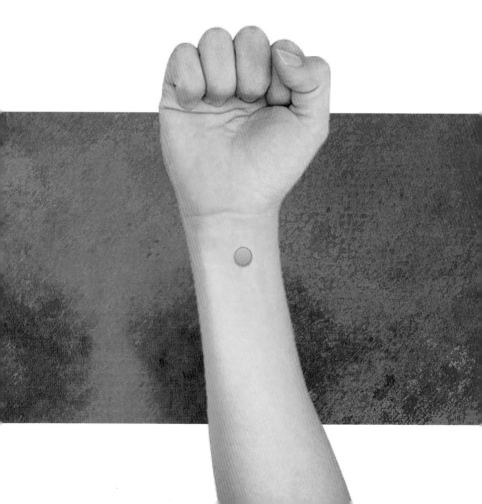

Triple Warmer Acupoint

Triple Warmer 5-Waiguan-Outer Pass

Location: Two thumb widths from wrist crease on midline of outer arm between the two bones.

Benefits: Fever, chills, headaches, neck strain, arm, elbow, wrist or finger problems, hand tremors, hearing issues or ringing in the ears.

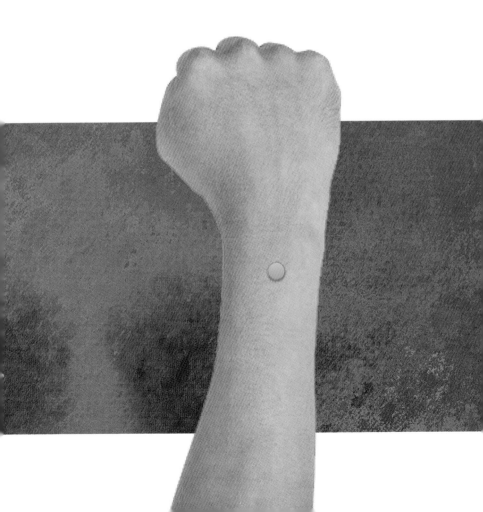

Time of Day Fire Meridians Peak

Energy travels in the acupuncture organs and meridians throughout the day in a 24-hour period.

Energy peaks in the heart channel at 11 AM to 1 PM.

12

1

2

I have heard that many heart attacks occur around noon. We are usually digesting lunch at 1 to 3 PM, so it is important to chew well, as the small intestine has no teeth and can only absorb small molecules of nutrition.

Energy peaks in the small intestine channel at 1 to 3 PM.

3

4

5

6

11

1

10

Energy peaks in the triple warmer at 9 to 11 PM.

9

Energy peaks in the pericardium channel at 7 to 9 PM.

8

7

Healing Sound for the Heart

Qigong has a healing sound for the major organs. *Ke* (pronounced *kurrrr*) is the sound for healing of the heart and easing heart fire.

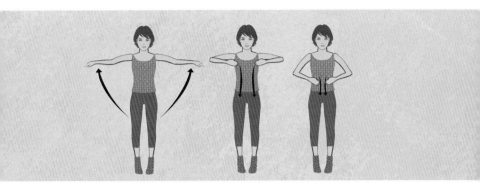

STEP 1: Inhale naturally and hold your breath. Raise both arms up from your side, your palms facing down. Relax your shoulders, keeping your wrists and elbows naturally bent and relaxed.

STEP 2: When your arms are even with your shoulders, rotate your palms until they are facing in and circle them toward your chest. Then, rotate your palms until the fingers of both hands are pointing at each other without touching and palms facing down. While holding your breath, imagine leading energy up from your left big toe up the inside of your left leg and into your abdomen. Continue up into your heart.

STEP 3: Exhale and vocalize the sound of *Ke* (*kurrrr*), (interestingly "coeur" is French for heart) with your mouth half open, tongue touching the bottom of your mouth, and exerting a slight pressure with your jaw. At the same time, lower both palms down to your abdomen. Hold up your anus area and draw your abdomen in. During exhalation, lead energy from your heart down the inside of your left arm to and out at the tip of your little finger. Exhale out all the impurities. Repeat steps 1 to 3 six times. This completes a set. Do three sets.

Taking Care
of the Heart

🔥 Align with your true nature and cultivate your own authenticity.

🔥 Have integrity in your relationships, knowing and expressing who you are and what you want.

🔥 Spend less time doing things that don't matter to you and with people who don't feed your spirit.

🔥 Meditation, prayer, drawing, journal writing, and mindful walking in nature nurture Shen.

As you balance your heart, your life is infused with a light or glow. You increase illumination, intuition, and insight into your everyday life, guiding your decisions. You will have greater ease in loving, discerning the differences between I and thou, and breaking patterns of codependency.

Five Elements Correspondence Chart

Element	Earth	Metal	Water	Wood	Fire
YIN ORGAN	Spleen	Lungs	Kidneys	Liver	Heart
YANG ORGAN	Stomach	Large Intestine	Bladder	Gallbladder	Small Intestine
BODY PART	Muscles	Skin	Bones and Joints	Tendons and Ligaments	Blood Vessels
COLOR	Yellow	White	Black	Green	Red
FACIAL DIAGNOSIS	Temples, Upper Lip	Cheeks, Lower Lip	Below Eyes, Chin	Between Eyebrows	Tip of Nose, Corners of Mouth
MERIDIAN PEAK TIME	7–11 AM	3–7 AM	3–7 PM	11 PM–3 AM	11AM–3 PM
ORIFICE	Mouth	Nose	Ears	Eyes	Tongue
PERIOD OF DAY	Afternoon	Sunset	Night	Morning	Midday
SEASON	Indian Summer	Fall	Winter	Spring	Summer
SENSE	Taste	Smell	Hearing	Vision	Speech
SPIRIT	Yi / Thought	Po / Corporeal Soul	Zhi / Will	Hun / Ethereal Soul	Shen / Spirit
TASTE	Sweet	Pungent / Hot	Salty	Sour	Bitter
WEATHER	Damp	Dry	Cold	Wind	Heat

Five Elements Symptom Chart

Earth	Metal	Water	Wood	Fire
Low blood sugar, hypoglycemia or diabetes	Tendency to get colds or coughs	Edema or swelling	Hasty or quick tempered	Insomnia
Bad digestion	Hay fever or other allergies	Pain in knees or ankles	Migraines	Palpitations
Abdominal pains or fullness	Asthma	Loss of sexual desire	Blurred vision	Cold extremities
Cold sores	Constipation or diarrhea	Urinate frequently or at night	Weak or breaking nails	Bright red or blotchy complexion or very pale
Spaced out, foggy headed	Itching or rashes	Lower back pain	Oily skin (especially around face, nose, and scalp)	Tendency to blush when nervous or upset
Energy goes up and down	Introverted	Overly cautious, avoids taking risks	Dry, red, itchy, or teary eyes	Spontaneous sweating, hot flashes, easily overheat
Thick mucus in nose, mouth, and throat	Dry hair or split ends	Darkish hue around or under eyes	Chronic tension in the neck and/or shoulders	Skin eruptions (acne, pimples, boils, rashes) that feel "hot" or inflamed
Gain weight easily, hard to lose weight	Sinus congestion	Teeth problems	Menstrual problems (cramping, irregular, with irritability or mood swings)	Varicose veins or hemorrhoids
Craving sweet and starchy foods	Moles or warts	Osteopenia or Osteoporosis	Tendency to have muscle and tendon injuries	Tongue problems (sores, inflammation, redness, swelling)
Gum issues (swollen, sore, receding, or bleeding)	Eczema or psoriasis	Hearing problems or ringing in ears	Heartburn	Speech problems (stammering, stuttering, slurring words, or speaking too quickly)

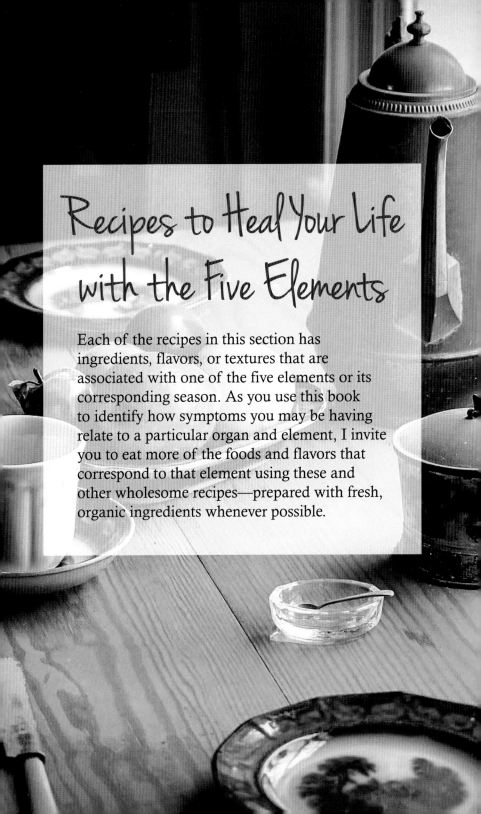

Recipes to Heal Your Life with the Five Elements

Each of the recipes in this section has ingredients, flavors, or textures that are associated with one of the five elements or its corresponding season. As you use this book to identify how symptoms you may be having relate to a particular organ and element, I invite you to eat more of the foods and flavors that correspond to that element using these and other wholesome recipes—prepared with fresh, organic ingredients whenever possible.

Earth Element
Carrot Squash Soup with Miso

2 onions, minced

2 carrots, cubed

1 kabocha, buttercup or butternut squash, peeled and cubed

1 tsp extra virgin olive oil

4–6 cups vegetable stock or water

1–2 tsp of light miso, or to taste

Parsley for garnish

1. Sauté onions with olive oil for about five minutes and add the rest of the vegetables and sauté for three minutes.

2. Add the vegetable stock or water and cook for about 20 minutes, or until vegetables are soft.

3. Dilute miso paste with water and add to soup and simmer on low heat for five minutes.

4. You can puree soup in a blender.

5. Serve in bowls and garnish each with a sprig of parsley.

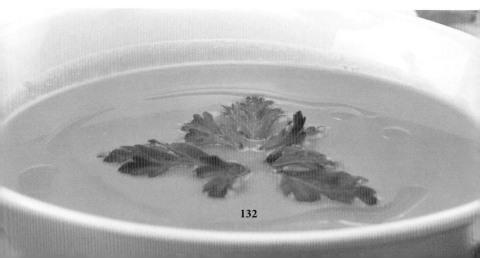

Earth Element
Creamy Millet

1 cup millet

1 cup mushrooms

1 cup onions

1 clove garlic, optional

2 cups purified water

Pinch of sea salt

1 quart-size pot

1. Wash the millet and soak overnight or for eight hours. (In the winter, lightly dry roast millet before soaking.)

2. Add the rinsed millet and purified water to a pot.

3. Cut mushrooms and onions into bite-size pieces.

4. Bring to boil, add the sea salt, then lower flame and simmer for about 30 minutes.

5. Serve porridge in bowls with a sprinkle of gomashio (sesame-sea salt condiment).

Option: For a delicious variation: cook the millet with other vegetables like cauliflower, squash, or carrots.

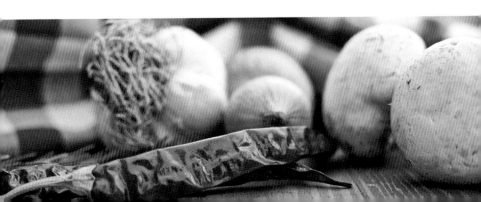

Earth Element
Sweet Vegetable Drink and Smoothie

½ cup onions

½ cup carrots

½ cup cabbage

½ cup sweet winter squash

8 cups purified water

1. Wash and finely chop or shred vegetables. In a pot add vegetables and water and bring to boil and then cover and simmer for 20 minutes. Don't add seasoning.

2. Strain vegetables and drink the juice warm. Store leftover in refrigerator, but heat again before using.

3. Add all remaining soft vegetables into a blender/mixer (after cooking) and mix until smooth. Drink warm or at room temperature as a smoothie.

This drink is beneficial for relaxing the body and muscles, softening the pancreas and helping to stabilize blood sugar levels. If you typically get a blood sugar drop in early afternoon, then drink a cup of the warm sweet liquid before that time and you should feel steady energy.

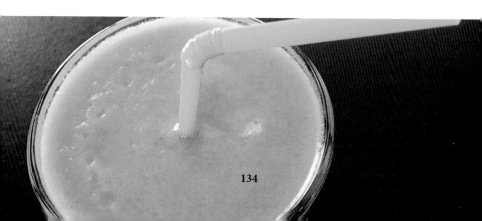

Earth Element

Gluten Free Almond Apple Crunch

4–5 baking apples

Lemon juice to coat the apples

½ cup raisins or other dried fruit, soaked and sliced

½ cup almond slivers, slightly toasted

1 tsp cinnamon

Pinch of sea salt

1 cup organic gluten free flour

2 cups gluten free whole grain rolled oats

½ cup oil (olive, coconut, safflower, sesame, grapeseed, or sunflower)

1 cup maple syrup

Filtered water, small amount

Preheat oven to 350° F.

1. Core four or five apples and cut into slices. Put in a baking dish and mix with lemon juice to stop oxidization. Add the soaked and sliced raisins, toasted nuts, cinnamon, and salt and mix.

2. In a separate bowl, mix the flour and rolled oats. Mix in the oil and maple syrup until you have small clumps. Spread evenly to cover the apples. Add a small amount of water to the pan and cover with parchment paper.

3. Bake covered for about 30 minutes and uncovered for about five minutes. Serve warm and top with Cashew Maple Whipped Cream (page 136).

Earth Element
Cashew Maple Whipped Cream

1 cup raw cashews

2 cups purified water

Vanilla extract to taste

Small pinch of sea salt

1 Tbsp maple syrup, or to taste

Garnish with sliced cashews

1. Soak one cup of cashews in two cups water overnight, and then drain. Reserve the soaking water.

2. Add nuts, vanilla, sea salt, and maple syrup to a blender or food processor and blend. Add in the soaking water until the desired creamy consistency is reached.

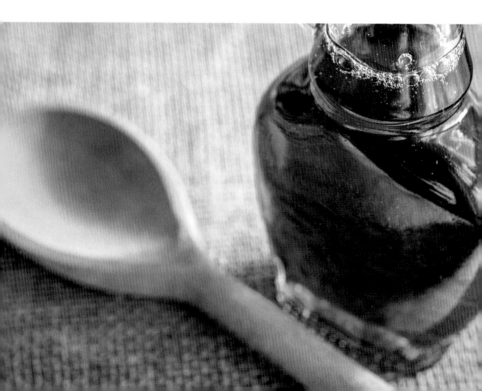

Metal Element

Green Leafy Vegetables with Caramelized Onions

1 Tbsp olive oil (or other healthy oil)

1 cup onion, finely diced

Seasoning: sea salt and pepper

2 cloves garlic, minced

1 smaller cauliflower, cut into small pieces

Purified/spring water

1 bunch collards or kale, or other greens

Garnish: chopped parsley

1. Wash and drain greens. Remove coarse stems and midribs. Cut into half-inch strips. Set aside. Cube the cauliflower. Peel and finely dice onions and garlic.

2. Heat the oil in a large skillet, add onions and sea salt and sauté them over medium-high heat until onions begin to brown, stirring constantly.

3. Add garlic, cauliflower, and a pinch of salt and pepper and stir for one minute. Half cover the vegetables with water and bring to a quick boil, then reduce heat and simmer until cauliflower is nearly done, for about five minutes.

4. Add greens and cook for five minutes more, or until all vegetables are done and water evaporates. Can add umeboshi plum vinegar or salt to taste.

5. Garnish with the chopped parsley.

Metal Element
Rice Pilaf

1 medium onion, chopped

1 medium green pepper, chopped

1 daikon radish (or 5 red radishes) sliced and cut into squares

1 Tbsp olive oil

1½ cups long grain brown rice, uncooked

2 garlic cloves, minced

1½ cups water

1 cup of vegetable or chicken broth

½ teaspoon dried thyme

¼ teaspoon black pepper

½ tsp fennel seeds

1. In large saucepan, sauté onion, daikon (or red) radish and green pepper in oil until tender.

2. Add rice and garlic; cook and stir for three to four minutes or until rice is lightly browned.

3. Add the water, broth, thyme, fennel seeds, and pepper.

4. Bring to a boil.

5. Reduce heat; cover and simmer for 35–40 minutes or until rice is tender.

6. Fluff with fork.

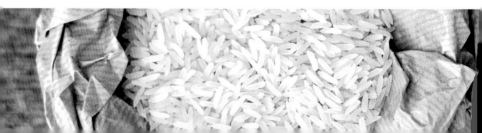

Metal Element
Sweet and Sour Chinese Cabbage

1 Tbsp extra virgin olive oil

1 medium red apple, cored and diced

1 medium sliced Chinese cabbage

1 daikon radish, sliced thin

1 tsp sea salt

1 tsp apple cider vinegar, or more to taste (or substitute balsamic or umeboshi plum vinegar)

Purified water

1. Heat oil in a stainless steel pot to medium heat. Add apple, and then cabbage, then daikon radish, stirring after each addition.

2. Add sea salt and apple cider vinegar and mix again.

3. Add water to half cover the vegetables. Bring all to a quick boil and simmer for about 10 minutes or until the cabbage is soft and tasty.

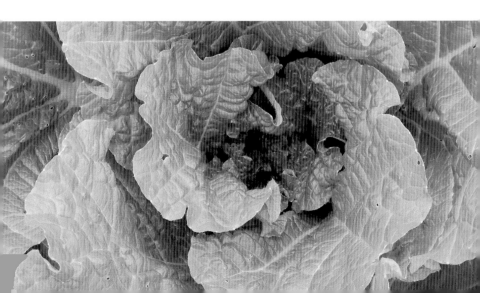

Metal Element
Curried Quinoa with Chickpeas

1½ cups water

½ cup orange juice

1 can chickpeas or garbanzo beans, rinsed and drained (or soak or cook beans from scratch)

2 medium tomatoes, seeded and chopped

1 medium sweet red pepper, julienned

1 cup quinoa, rinsed

2 stalks sliced celery

1 small red onion, finely chopped

½ cup raisins

1 tsp curry powder

1 tsp ginger powder or fresh grated ginger

½ cup minced fresh cilantro

1. In a large saucepan, bring water and orange juice to a boil. Stir in chickpeas, tomatoes, red pepper, celery, quinoa, onion, raisins, ginger, and curry. Return to a boil. Reduce heat; cover and simmer for 15–20 minutes or until liquid is absorbed.

2. Remove from heat; fluff with a fork. Sprinkle with cilantro.

3. Option: Cooked brown rice can be used in place of quinoa; just increase the total cooking time to 45 minutes.

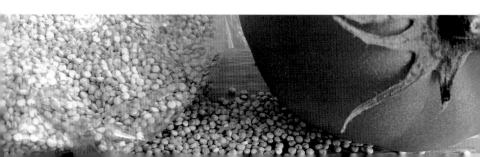

Water Element
Miso Soup with Seaweed

4 cups of purified water

2–3 shiitake mushroom, soaked and cut

1 small piece of kombu sea vegetable

½ cup onions, sliced into thin half-moons

½ strip of wakame, broken into pieces

2 carrots sliced and quartered

4 tsp brown rice miso (or other miso), to taste, diluted with a little bit of warm water

Scallions for garnish (or parsley)

1. Boil water, kombu, and shiitake for 10 minutes. Remove the kombu and cut into bite-size pieces and return. Add the vegetables and simmer for five minutes or until soft, and then add the wakame.

2. Dilute the miso with a little bit of warm water and add to the soup. Simmer, not boil, for three minutes.

3. Serve and garnish with chopped scallions.

Option to add any veggies you like such as kale, broccoli, cauliflower, or root vegetables.

You may also add an egg toward the end and make like egg drop soup for extra protein.

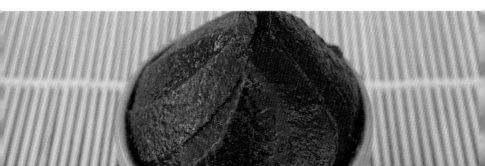

Water Element
Carrot and Burdock Kinpira

1 cup burdock root

2 cups carrots

1 tsp light sesame oil

Purified water

2 Tbsp tamari or soy sauce, or to taste

2 big pinches of arame or hijiki seaweed, soaked until soft

1. Wash burdock and carrots with a vegetable brush and cut into diagonal ovals, then into matchsticks.

2. Heat oil in frying pan. Add the burdock and sauté for a couple of minutes and then add carrots and sauté both for two to three minutes.

3. Add a small amount of water to half cover the vegetables. Add tamari or soy sauce to taste. Bring to boil, reduce heat, cover, and simmer for about 30 minutes.

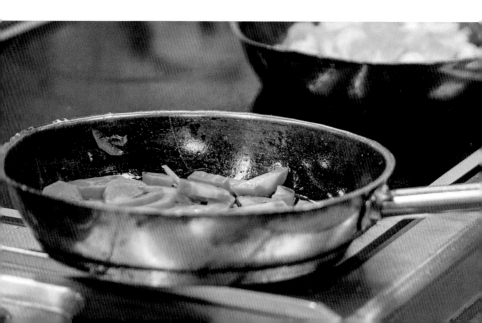

Water Element
Red Rice

2 cups organic short grain brown rice

⅓ cup azuki or red beans

2 cups of filtered or spring water per cup of rice

2-inch piece of kombu sea vegetable (to cut down on gas from beans)

1. Wash and then soak rice and beans overnight or for six to eight hours.

2. Discard soaking water and replace the same amount of fresh water.

3. Place the rice, beans, kombu, and fresh water in a heavy pot. Bring to a boil, and scoop up some of the foam and replace with purified water.

4. Cover the pot and simmer on very low heat for 60 minutes. Then remove from heat and let the rice rest in the pot for about five minutes, then mix and scoop it into a bowl to serve.

Or for softer and more digestible dish, try pressure-cooking.

Place rice, beans, kombu, and water in a pressure cooker. Bring to a boil, and scoop up some of the foam and replace with a little purified water. Fasten down the cover and when the pressure is high, reduce the flame to medium low. Pressure-cook the rice for 45 minutes. Remove from heat and let the pressure completely cool down before taking off the cover. Mix and serve.

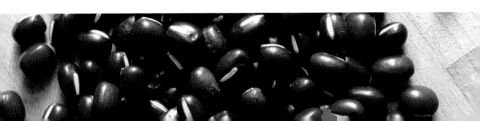

Water Element
Black Beans and Carrots

1 cup black beans

3 cups water

2-inch piece of kombu sea vegetable

$\frac{1}{8}$ tsp sea salt per cup of beans

1½ tsp tamari or soy sauce

1 cup carrots, cubed

½ cup cilantro, shopped

1. Wash beans with cold water, add water and soak for eight hours or overnight.

2. Use three cups of fresh water, add kombu, and bring to a boil and then simmer about three hours, or till soft. Check the water level occasionally. Toward the end of cooking add sea salt, tamari, and carrots.

3. Simmer for 5 to 15 minutes before serving.

4. Garnish with chopped cilantro.

For pressure-cooking.

1. Pressure-cook the beans for about one hour. Release the pressure and add sea salt, tamari to taste, and the carrots.

2. Simmer for 5 to 15 minutes before serving.

Optional: Use other vegetables like squash or onions and add spices like ginger, turmeric, or chili pepper.

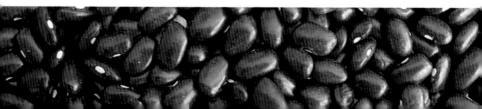

Wood Element
Crunchy Mung Bean Sprouts Salad with Green Olives

2 cups napa or Chinese cabbage

½ cup spring carrots, julienne, grated, or matchstick-cut

1 cup mung bean sprouts

¾ cup pitted green olives, sliced

3 scallions, both the green and white parts, finely sliced

Lemon or lime juice, to taste

1 tsp tamari

1 tsp extra virgin olive oil

1. Slice cabbage into one-inch slices.

2. Place the carrots, scallions, mung bean sprouts, and sliced green olives into a mixing bowl.

3. Add lemon or lime juice, oil, and tamari, and mix, pressing and squeezing all gently with your hands. Serve raw.

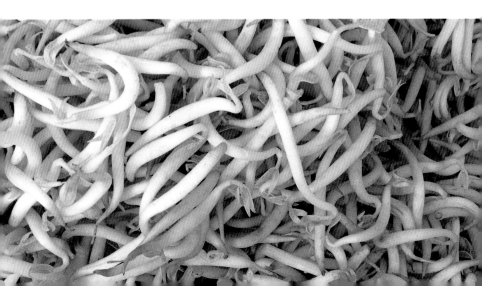

Wood Element
Barley Soup with Mushrooms and Scallions

½ cup barley

Scallions, finely sliced

1 cup mushrooms, sliced

1 cup celery, sliced

5 cups water

1 heaping Tbsp of miso paste

1. Wash barley and soak for six to eight hours or overnight. After soaking rinse and replace water.

2. Slice mushrooms and celery. Add mushrooms and celery to barley with water. Boil until barley is soft, about 1.5 hours.

3. Dissolve miso in stew broth and simmer for five minutes. Garnish each bowl of soup with sliced scallions.

Optional: Add any other vegetables you like such as red cabbage or turnips.

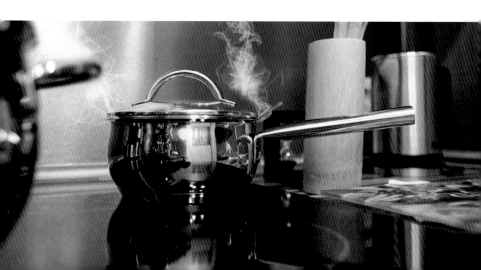

Wood Element
Lemony Lima Beans Dip

2 cups lima beans, cooked, or can of beans

1 inch of kombu sea vegetable

1 tsp sea salt per cup of beans

1 Tbsp of tamari, or to taste

2 Tbsp lemon juice, or to taste

2 cloves garlic, crushed

1 Tbsp sesame tahini or other nut butter

1. Wash and soak beans overnight. Strain and replace with fresh filtered water.

2. Boil lima beans with kombu until soft, then add sea salt and cook for seven more minutes.

3. Mash with a potato masher or in a food processor until smooth.

4. Add tamari and lemon juice to taste. Use as a dip with vegetables or crackers or as a spread.

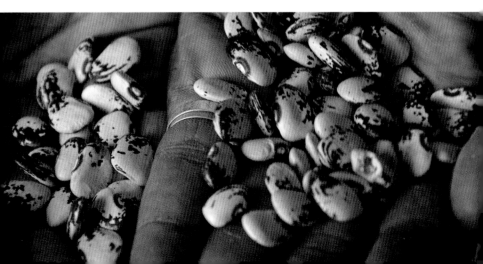

Wood Element
Apple Cider Vinegar Dressing

½ cup apple cider vinegar

½ cup olive oil

¼ teaspoon sea salt or Himalayan salt

¼ teaspoon pepper

1 clove garlic, finely minced

2 Tbsp honey

Optional: 1 Tbsp Dijon mustard

Add all ingredients to a jar with a lid and shake vigorously to combine.

Optional: Use brown rice vinegar or umeboshi plum vinegar.

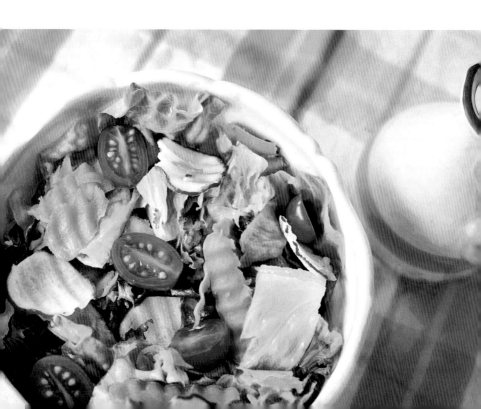

Fire Element
Fruit Salad with Ginger and Mint

1 pint raspberries

1 pint blueberries

1 pint strawberries, if big, cut in half

1 small pineapple, peeled and diced

1 Tbsp ginger, finely grated

1 lemon, juiced

1 orange, juiced

Pinch of sea salt

½ cup mint, finely minced

Place fruit in a bowl. Squeeze the finely grated ginger over the fruit, and squeeze the juice from the ginger pulp into a smaller bowl. Add the juice of one lemon and one small orange, add the sea salt, and mix. Gently toss the dressing with the fruit and cool for several hours. Serve cold and garnish with the finely minced mint.

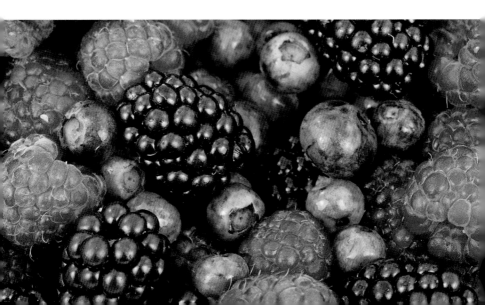

Fire Element
Avocado Salsa

2.5 cucumbers, peeled, seeded, and diced

1 cup red onions, chopped

2 small jalapenos, seeded and chopped

3 avocados, ripe but not too soft, sliced

½ cup cilantro leaves, finely chopped

Dressing

3½ Tbsp extra virgin olive oil

3 Tbsp lime juice, freshly squeezed

2 cloves garlic, finely minced

½ tsp sea salt, or to taste

¼ tsp ground pepper, freshly ground

1. Rinse chopped onions under cold water to remove the harsh bite and then drain well. In a bowl, add the cucumbers, onions, jalapenos, and avocados.

2. Mix the dressing with a whisk and pour over the cucumber and avocado and gently toss, adding the cilantro.

3. Serve with organic chips, crackers, or veggies or as a side dish.

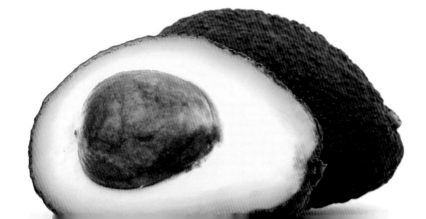

Fire Element
Quinoa with Summer Vegetables

¾ cup quinoa, yellow

1½ cups of water

Pinch sea salt

1 small zucchini

1 cup Chinese cabbage

¾ cup of hard tofu, cubed, or cooked chickpeas

1 Tbsp wheat free tamari, to taste

2 cloves minced garlic

Juice from ½ lemon or lime

½ Tbsp ginger

½ Tbsp turmeric

Cayenne pepper to taste

1. Wash quinoa and strain. Bring quinoa and water to a boil, lower flame, add sea salt and seasonings to taste, and simmer for 20 minutes. Fluff and set aside.

2. Water sauté the vegetables and the tofu and seasoning with tamari. Combine quinoa, tofu, and vegetables. Serve on a raw Chinese cabbage leaf.

Add other summer vegetables like mustard greens, watercress, or mushrooms. If you are sensitive to soy, substitute tofu with cooked chickpeas and tamari with soy free and wheat free coconut aminos sauce.

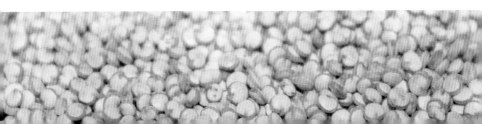

Fire Element
Blanched Greens

2 types of greens (kale, mustard greens, watercress, swiss chard, collard greens)

1 leek, sliced

2 Tbsp olive oil

2 tsp brown rice vinegar or umeboshi plum vinegar

Cayenne pepper

1. Cut the greens into slices and bite-size pieces. Boil a pot of water and put in greens and cover and let simmer for two to three minutes.

2. Remove veggies and strain off water.

3. Mix in the olive oil and brown rice vinegar or umeboshi plum vinegar.

4. Add pinches of cayenne pepper to taste.

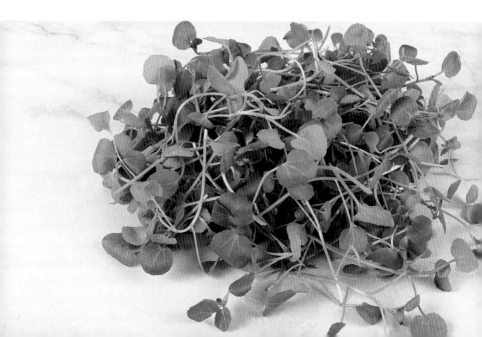

Timely Tips to Toxin-Proof Your Life

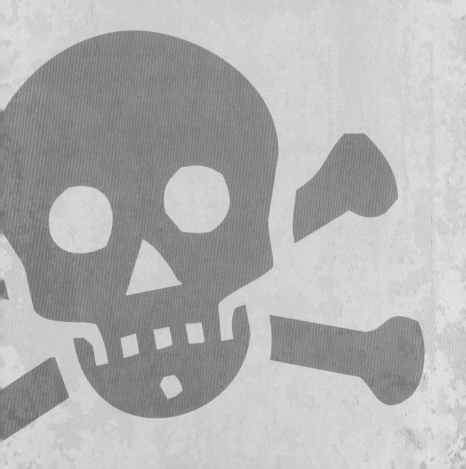

I had a teenage patient complaining of a tight chest and rapid heartbeat. She noticed it only happened on weekdays, always after a school lunch. She always had what she thought was the healthiest choice, a salad. When she brought her own organic lunch to school, the symptoms disappeared.

Lettuce

Many of us want to choose a healthy meal, so we often go for salads. Be careful though because vegetables that are not organic can have traces of pesticides. So get organic when possible.

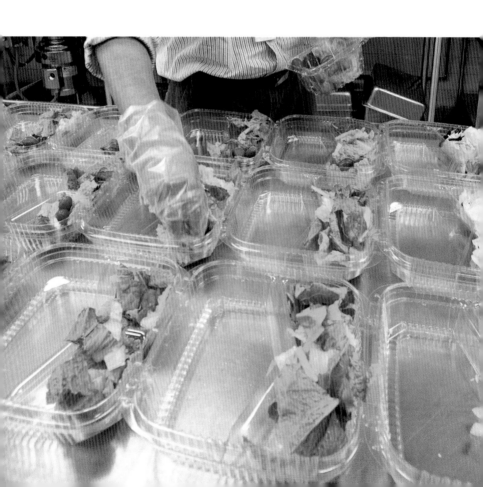

Cord Blood Study

In 2004, Environmental Working Group (EWG) tested cord blood of 10 newborns and found an average of 204 chemicals per baby. A total of 287 different chemicals were found.

- 180 cause cancer.
- 217 are toxic to the brain and nervous system.
- 208 cause birth defects or abnormal development in animal studies.

There has been a dramatic rise in autism, Parkinson's, and Alzheimer's over the last 20 years, which is likely made worse by toxins.

The EWG only tested for a few hundred out of a possible 90,000 chemicals, so they would have found more if they had tested for them. It cost $10,000 per child to do the testing.

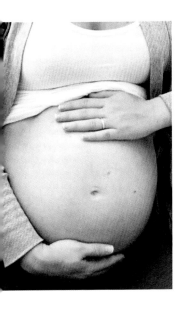

Some of these chemicals, like nonstick chemicals used in clothes, furniture, food wrappers, and nonstick pans, even showed up in penguins and Arctic seagulls.

Toxins bioaccumulate, meaning that those at the top of the food chain get the most concentrated chemicals.

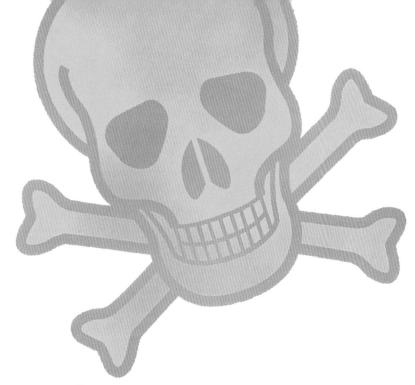

Process of Disease

1. Absorption of toxins

2. Deposition of toxins

3. Degeneration by toxins

The body will try to expel toxins with vomiting, fever, diarrhea, and/or skin rash.

Some toxins are from within the body (like from food allergies, parasites, yeast, poor digestion), and some are from the outside.

In "Timely Tips to Toxin-Proof Your Life," we are focusing on external toxins.

Toxins

Toxins block the function of mitochondria, the cells' energy centers. This can cause fatigue. The recent rise of autoimmune diseases reflects the increase of toxicity in the environment.

Most environmental toxins are fat soluble. The liver processes foods and transforms them from being fat soluble to water soluble so they can be eliminated.

Becoming obese may be a sign of toxicity. The body's intelligence may be storing toxins away from major organs because it can't find a way to eliminate them.

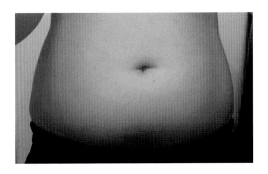

Chronic Toxicity Symptoms

- Fatigue
- Sleep disturbance
- Intestinal distress
- Allergies
- Headaches
- Confusion
- Anxiety

Pesticides

More than five billion pounds of pesticides are used in the United States every year.

More than 20,000 pesticides are registered with the Environmental Protection Agency.

Pesticides are used on livestock to control insects and are in their feed as well.

Pesticides are the most common environmental toxin I see affecting people. You need to eat mostly organic, especially for the dirty dozen. Eating at restaurants frequently is a real risk.

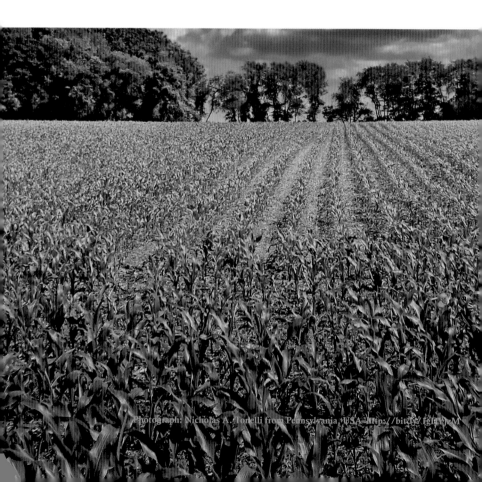

Photograph: Nicholas A. Tonelli from Pennsylvania, USA http://bit.ly/1glnWyM

The Dirty Dozen

The dirty dozen are the fruits and vegetables with the highest pesticide residues.

1. Strawberries

2. Spinach

3. Kale

4. Nectarines

5. Apples

6. Grapes

7. Peaches

8. Cherries

9. Pears

10. Tomatoes

11. Celery

12. Potatoes

The Clean 15

These are the fruits and vegetables that have the least amount of pesticide residue. So if you can't afford to buy everything organic or you are eating out, these are the ones to go for.

1. Avocados

2. Sweet corn

3. Pineapples

4. Sweet peas (frozen)

5. Onions

6. Papayas

7. Eggplants

8. Asparagus

9. Kiwis

10. Cabbage

11. Cauliflower

12. Cantaloupes

13. Broccoli

14. Mushrooms

15. Honeydew

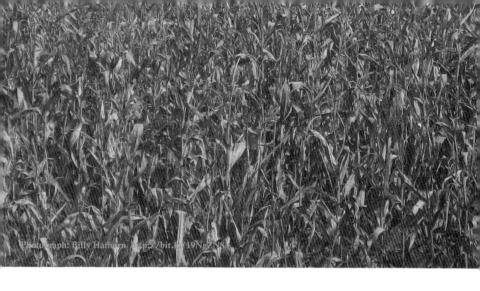

Pesticides and GMOs

The average child in the United States between the ages of 6 and 11 has been found to have four times the acceptable levels of pesticides in their systems. This may correspond with many childhood diseases that are on the rise.

Now GMO plants like corn produce a pesticide in every cell of the plant.

This pesticide, or Bt toxin, has been found in 93% of pregnant women and 80% of umbilical blood of babies. This can create learning problems, allergies, digestive problems, and autoimmune diseases.

I have noticed, as have other healers, that many patients who feel unwell even though they eat a very limited and strict diet, go to Europe and eat a rich, gluten-full, wide diet and feel great and then feel poorly when back in the US even when eating healthy food.

Genetically Modified (GM) Crops

Some crops are genetically engineered to withstand herbicides such as Roundup®. This has led to an increased use of chemicals and the development of resistant super weeds that nothing can kill.

- 88% of soybeans
- 91% of corn
- 100% canola oil

About 70% of processed foods contain GM ingredients.

Animals get fatter when fed GM corn...and so do we.

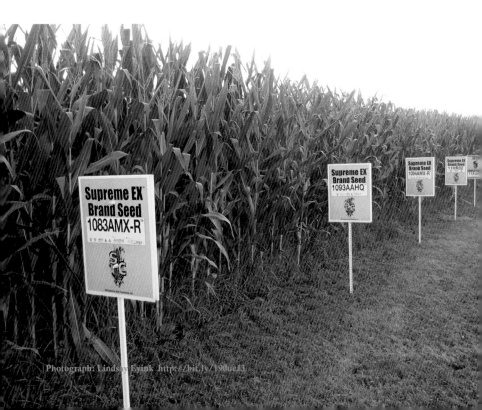

Are Organic Foods Better for You?

Commercial vegetables are larger than they used to be, but **have 5–40% fewer minerals, such as magnesium, iron, calcium, and zinc, than 50 years ago…and they aren't as tasty.**

Healthier soil leads to higher levels of nutrients in crops.

Children with higher levels of pesticides had a higher risk of ADHD.

Organic fruits and vegetables have 40% more antioxidants. Organic milk has 90% more.

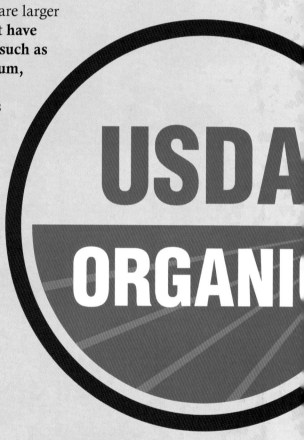

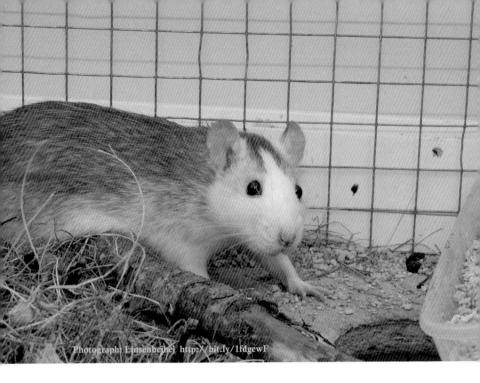

Rats and Organics

In 2005, scientists compared the health of rats fed conventional diets to those on organic diets. Rats fed organic foods had the following.

- Improved immune system status.
- Better sleeping habits.
- Less weight and slimmer appearance.
- Higher vitamin E content in their blood.

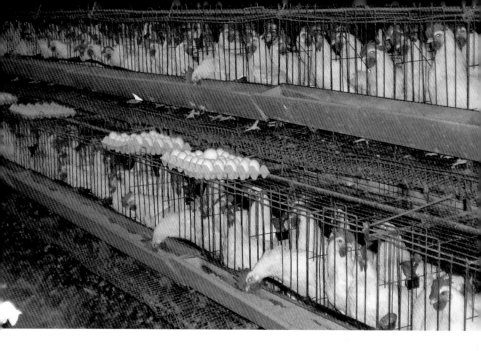

Animal Foods

Grazing and growing feed for livestock uses 70% of all agricultural land and 30% of the earth's land surface.

CAFOs: (concentrated animal feeding operation)

- Produce enormous amounts of sewage, methane, and other pollutants.

- Can house hundreds to millions of animals.

They are not the image of farms that we grew up with. These are animal concentration camps. Egg-laying machine chickens are stacked in cages, unable to move. Hogs are housed in cages where they can't even turn around, biting at the metal bars as they go insane. Cows are now fed GMO corn and soy instead of grass, which their digestive tracts are not made to digest.

Animal Products

Turkeys are often so cramped that they will peck each other to death, and as a result their beaks can be cut off.

Animals that like to be clean are caked in their own waste.

Many animals are diseased, and have a continuous feeding of antibiotics, hormones, and pesticide-laden grain, which all end up in the milk, meat, and eggs.

Hormones are used to make larger animals or produce more milk.

Animals are often cut open while still alive, and all that pain and suffering is part of the meat you eat.

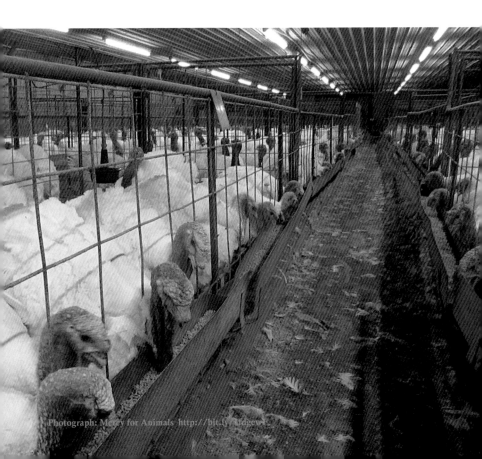

Photograph: Mercy for Animals http://bit.ly/tfdgcw

Bred to Be Huge!

Look at this image showing how we have bred chickens to become gigantic in a much shorter time span. Some cannot even walk. If we eat this kind of food often, it's no surprise that our children become obese at younger and younger ages. The hormones, antibiotics, and arsenic fed to them to make them fat can do the same to us.

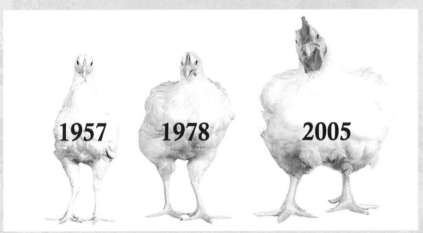

Photograph: Poultry Science

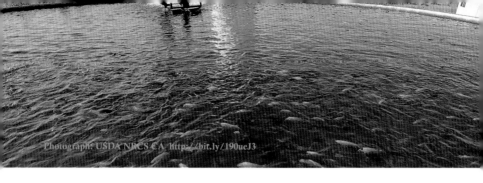

Farmed Fish

About 84% of seafood in the United States is imported, and half of that is farm raised.

Every Atlantic salmon must eat five times its weight in fish. To save on fish, they are now eating barley, corn, and soybeans, not their native diet.

Fish feed contains chemicals and antibiotics as well to deal with health issues from overcrowding and filth.

Common environmental toxins like dioxins and PCBs are seven times higher in farmed than wild fish, which have high levels of toxicity already.

Salmon are not supposed to be kept in pens like couch potatoes. They are supposed to swim up rivers and waterfalls. Sitting around eating all day to get fat quickly is what they do, and that is what happens to those who eat them.

Now the fish industry wants to genetically engineer salmon with an eel-like fish to produce a creature that is twice as big as a normal salmon and matures in half the time.

You are what you eat!

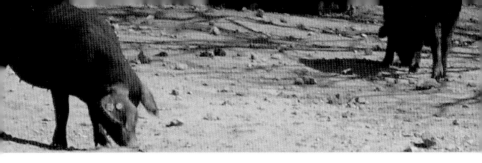

Humanely Raised Animals

If you decide to eat animal foods, vote with your pocketbook.

Animals should have space to do what they like to do in nature.

They should eat what they eat in nature. Cows like grass and pasture, not genetically modified corn and soy.

They should be killed by the quickest and most painless methods possible.

Chickens like to peck and scratch the ground and look for insects. Pigs like to root around on the ground. Some studies suggest they are smarter than dogs.

> *I saw one study where a dog and pig were trained to use a computer joystick and when they scored they got food. The pig was able to do it every time after it learned how. The dog had to be retaught every time.*

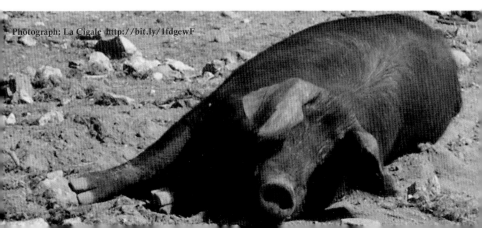

Preservatives

Preservatives keep food from going bad.

There are time-tested methods, such as using salt, vinegar, sugar, and ascorbic acid.

But today, **most preservatives are synthetic and toxic and tumor causing.**

They prevent bacterial, mold, and yeast growth, preserve color and flavor, and keep foods fresh by preventing oxidation and rancidity.

Most chemical preservatives affect the nervous system, and some have an impact on reproductive health or weaken the immune system.

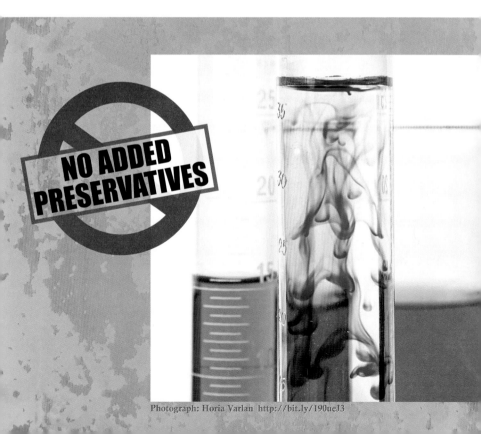

Photograph: Horia Varlan http://bit.ly/190ueJ3

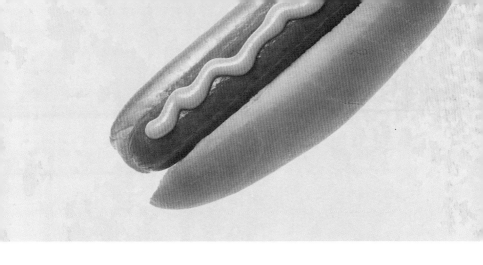

Modern Preservatives

Nitrates enhance flavor and preserve color, mostly in meats. **They are carcinogenic and should be avoided, especially for children.**

Sulfites and sulfur dioxide are derived from coal tar. They keep food from browning and are found in dried fruit and wine and can cause headaches, hyperactivity, and asthma.

BHA and BHT are considered the most dangerous preservatives and are outlawed in many other countries. They are carcinogens and have been found to cause stomach cancer. Baby mice exposed to these preservatives weighed less, slept less, and fought more. Although these preservatives are found in low levels in an individual food, over the years they accumulate and can cause serious problems.

Benzoic acid and sodium benzoate are found in many products and also cause hyperactivity and can cause eye and skin irritation. They are found in acidic foods like dressings, carbonated drinks, pickles, condiments, and jams and jellies.

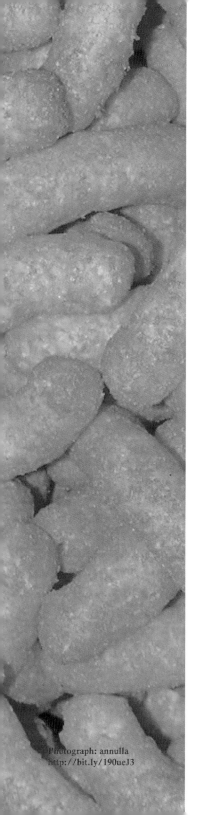

Artificial Colors

**One of the most widely used and
dangerous additives.**

In Europe, warning labels are
required on foods with dyes, but not
in the United States.

Many dyes cause tumor growth
in rodents and some create
hyperactivity in children.

Every year, food manufacturers
pour 15 million pounds of artificial
food dyes into US foods.

*I notice that most parents don't think
twice about giving their children
rainbow-colored cereal or fluorescent-
blue drinks and slushies, and they don't
consider bright orange cheese puffs out
of the ordinary, either. But the same
people often make sure their pets are
eating all-natural dog food.*

Blue #1 causes kidney cancer in mice.

Blue #2 also causes cancer, especially brain tumors in male rats.

Citrus red #2 is found in Florida orange skins and causes bladder cancer in rodents.

Green #2 causes increase in bladder and testes tumors in male rats, but at least your prescription drugs have a nice color!

Red #3, the dye that makes maraschino cherries bright red, has been recognized as a thyroid carcinogen by the FDA since 1990.

Red #40 is the most commonly consumed dye and may accelerate immune system tumors and cause allergies and hyperactivity.

Yellow #5 can cause hyperactivity and other behavioral changes in children.

Yellow #6 causes adrenal tumors and severe reactions in some people.

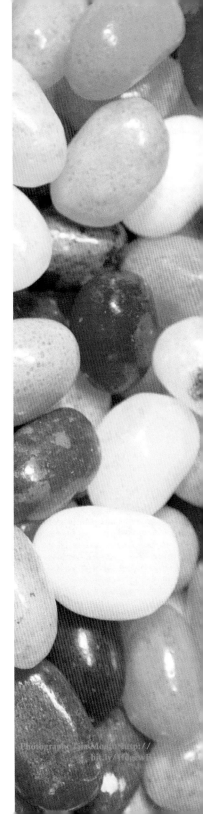

173

Monosodium glutamate (MSG) is added to food to enhance flavor. It produces many symptoms in sensitive people.

MSG is a form of concentrated salt added to foods to enhance the flavor.

It is particularly harmful to the nerves and brain and may be linked to Alzheimer's and Parkinson's diseases.

It's dangerous because it can cause these symptoms.

- Migraine headaches
- Balance difficulties
- Disabling arthritis
- Serious depression
- Behavioral problems in children
- Severe shortness of breath, asthma attacks, and heart irregularities

MSG is a very toxic substance, particularly to the developing brain, especially in the developing fetus.

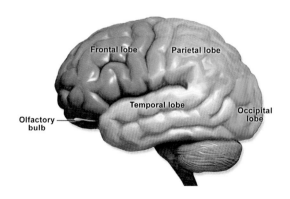

Image: Blausen.com staff. "Blausen gallery 2014." Wikiversity Journal of Medicine. DOI:10.15347/wjm/2014.010. ISSN 20018762

The amount of MSG used in food has doubled every decade since it was first used in the 1940s.

It is hidden in many foods under innocuous-sounding names. The food industry tends to rename MSG to avoid public scrutiny. There are approximately 40 names for it, including the words "hydrolyzed" or "autolyzed" yeast or "yeast extract." It may be derived from a fermented protein like soy protein or whey protein.

Under current FDA regulations, when MSG is added to a food, it must be identified as monosodium glutamate in the label's ingredient list. However, if MSG is part of a spice mix that is purchased by another company, the manufacturer does not have to list the ingredients of that spice mix and may use the words "flavorings" or "spices."

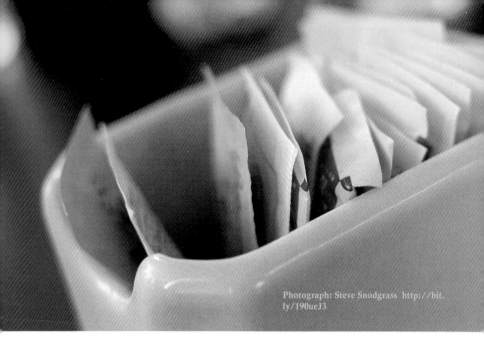

Artificial Sweeteners

Artificial sweeteners are now found in thousands of products and should be avoided.

Being around 200 times sweeter than sugar, artificial sweeteners negatively affect blood sugar and create more sweet cravings. Nobody really loses weight on these products.

These sweeteners trick the body into thinking that carbs are coming, so the pancreas releases insulin, causing a yo-yo effect in the blood sugar.

They also make you used to food being so sweet that you can't taste the subtle sweetness found in vegetables and grains.

Artificial sweeteners have been found to throw off the balance of bacteria in the intestines, leading to diabetes and weight gain, the exact things people who take them are trying to avoid.

NutraSweet®, or **aspartame,** has had the most reported adverse effects, largely on the nervous system. It is transformed into formaldehyde in the body and has been found in the liver, kidneys, and brains of those who consume it. It can also affect vision. It is called an excitotoxin because it stimulates nerve and brain cells to the point that they may die.

Acesulfame K, brand names Sunett® and Sweet One®, is the least studied and may cause cancer and damage to the organs, so it is best to avoid it.

Sucralose or **Splenda®** is a denatured sugar that has added chlorine. It has been shown to shrink the thymus, which I find is a key to immunity and fighting cancer. It damages the liver and kidneys and reduces the beneficial bacteria, which is a key to immunity and digestive health.

Saccharine or **Sweet'N Low®** used to have a warning for bladder cancer, which has been removed, but it is really not safe to use.

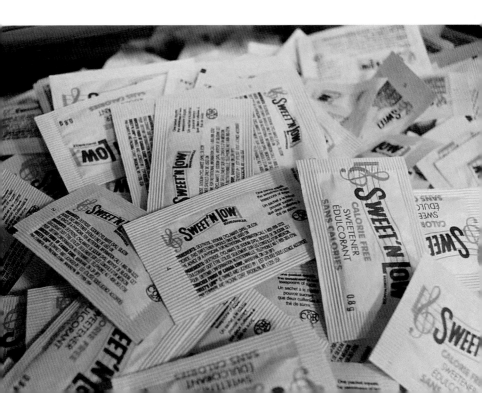

Fluoride

Fluoride is found in 70% of our water supply.

There is no difference between rates of tooth decay in fluoridated and non-fluoridated water.

The level of fluoride in tap water is 250 times the level found in breast milk.

Fluoride is a byproduct of fertilizer manufacturing and is contaminated with lead, arsenic, and aluminum.

Fluoride lowers the IQ of children.

Reverse osmosis removes fluoride from the water. Most other filters do not.

Cities are starting to decide to save money and people's health by stopping fluoridation. Some cities have lowered the fluoride level because children were getting permanently mottled teeth.

When I go to the dentist, I have them polish my teeth with pumice and I forgo the fluoride treatments.

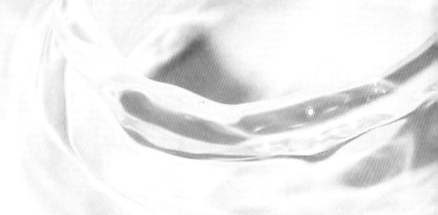

Tap Water and Chlorine

The chlorine in tap water combines with organic matter in the water and creates chlorine disinfection byproducts, which are potent carcinogens.

Chlorine kills bacteria, including beneficial flora in the intestines. It can also cause bone loss, allergies, asthma, birth defects, and hardening of the arteries.

Drugs are found in tap water from urine, which doesn't filter them out.

Fish are having their sex changed from birth control pills entering the water. In studies, half of all male fish were making eggs in one river, and one-fourth had damaged sperm. This may be responsible for the rise in human infertility.

Drink and cook only with filtered or spring water.

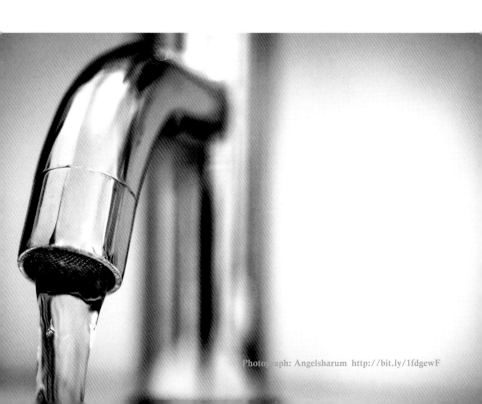

Mercury

Dental fillings are often called "silver fillings," but they are more than 50% mercury. The mercury constantly off-gasses and accumulates in the body.

If one filling was dissolved in a 10-acre lake, there would be an advisory not to eat fish from that lake.

Mercury is also found in many fish. This is often caused by waste from the burning of coal for energy, which ends up in lakes and rivers.

The new fluorescent light bulbs contain mercury as well.

The most serious and hard-to-treat diseases are very often from the mercury in dental fillings.

Some very bad cases of eczema and psoriasis have been cured after removing mercury and detoxifying the body.

Mercury should be illegal to use in dentistry.

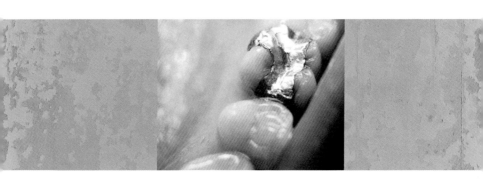

I had a patient who thought she had multiple sclerosis.
I found that it was actually mercury poisoning from fish. She
had been in Florida and eaten grouper every day. More mercury
bioaccumulates when larger fish eat smaller fish.

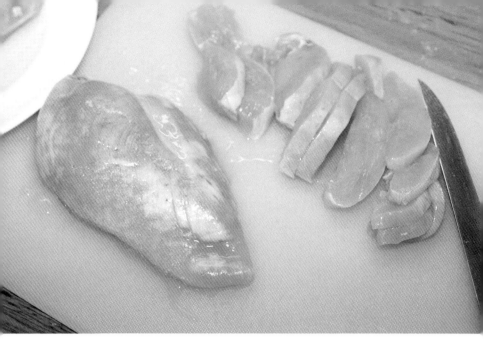

Arsenic

Treated wood used to be a source of arsenic.

Now arsenic is fed to commercial chickens to make them grow bigger and give them a pink color. Arsenic kills parasites so the chickens grow larger. It damages their blood vessels, giving the meat a pinker color.

Levels in chickens are six to nine times higher than the maximum level allowed in drinking water, and chicken litter is now fed to cows! One farmer in Arkansas spread chicken litter on his land, and arsenic started showing up in the houses nearby.

Now rice is showing up high in arsenic. Some of it is in the soil where they used to grow cotton, which was treated with pesticides that contained arsenic.

Aluminum

Aluminum is toxic to the nervous system. It is found in cookware, aluminum foil, deodorants and antiperspirants, table salt, vaccines, and aluminum cans.

The outer breast near the underarm is where most breast cancers occur, leading some to surmise that antiperspirants may play a role in breast cancer. Aluminum shows up concentrated in the brains of Alzheimer's patients.

I prefer stainless steel, ceramic, and enamel-coated cookware.

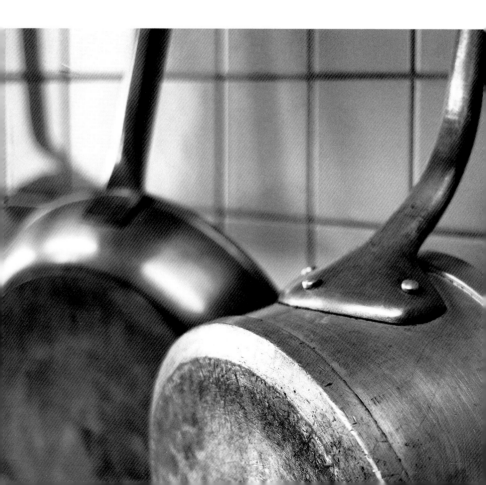

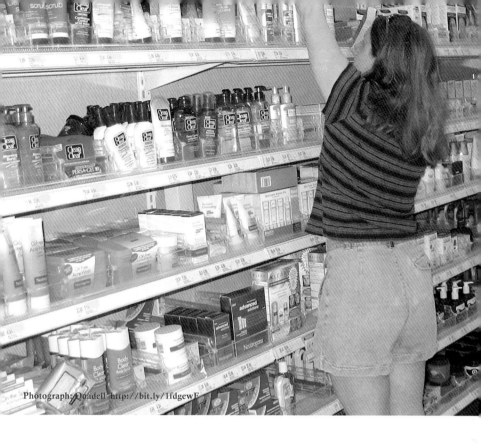

Personal Care Products

A person is exposed to 126 chemicals a day through personal care products.

Phthalate plasticizers, paraben preservatives, the antibiotic triclosan, synthetic musks, and sunscreen can disrupt hormones.

The Environmental Working Group has a cosmetics database called Skin Deep®, which lets you search over 75,000 ingredients for safety.

NBC TV Producer Did Her Own Experiment

A producer for *Dateline NBC* took urine tests for herself and her two children for BPA, phthalates, and triclosan, "the deadly three." These chemicals have been found in 90% of the population.

Her levels were high on the tests. Her six-month-old baby had 10 times the average of triclosan (an antibiotic found in antibiotic soaps), and her toddler had 100 times the average. These chemicals are found in hand soaps, canned foods, cash register receipts, paper money, plastic containers, and more. Hormone disrupters like bisphenol A can cause childhood obesity, ADD, autism, and infertility.

Levels of these chemicals went way down when the family ate organic foods and used natural beauty and cleaning products. They skyrocketed again when the producer intentionally went back to her old ways of microwaving, drinking diet soda, and using toxic products to see if the test results would go back up.

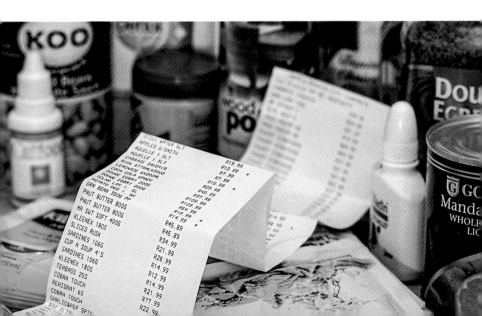

EMFs

EMFs (electromagnetic fields) are a new source of toxicity for many people. Cell phone towers, cell phones, computers, Wi-Fi, Bluetooth, cordless phones, electrical appliances, and wiring can interfere with the body's cells, signaling, and communication.

EMFs can lower immunity, melatonin, thyroid and testosterone levels. And they accelerate the growth of mold and viruses.

- A teenager had a cyst on his pituitary gland that was from a wire in his mouth, along with hours a day spent playing video games with a Bluetooth headset.

- A woman who kept her cell phone in her bra developed a breast tumor in the shape of a rectangle.

Every week I have to tell a few people that they are being affected by Wi-Fi and they should at least turn it off while they sleep. I advise people to keep cell phones out of their bedrooms while sleeping. I rewired my whole house to get rid of EMFs.

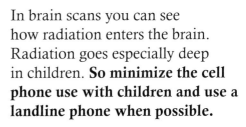

Cell Phones

In brain scans you can see how radiation enters the brain. Radiation goes especially deep in children. **So minimize the cell phone use with children and use a landline phone when possible.**

It is best to keep your cell phone off your body when you're not using it and use it as a speakerphone to keep it away from your brain.

Cell phones have been shown to have a link to DNA damage, along with these problems.

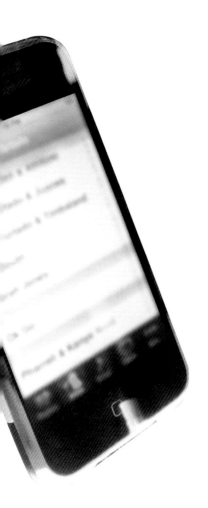

- Memory loss
- Alzheimer's disease
- Cancer
- Breakdown of the brain's defenses
- Reduced sperm count

When reception is bad and you have only a few bars, the phone must send out a stronger signal. **Keep your cell phone away from your body when it's on. It is best to limit cell phone usage to brief messages, texting, and short conversations.**

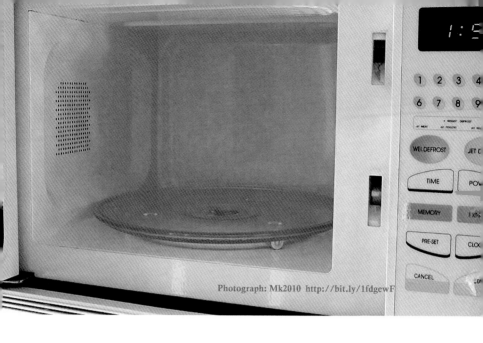

Microwaves

Plastic containers or tableware can leach into the food. Plastics can mimic estrogen in the body and create health problems.

Microwaves can damage food on a molecular level. Microwaves destroy the energetic level of foods by 60%–90%, and harm the vitamins, minerals, and enzymes in the food.

Some research says there has been more tumor formation especially in the stomach and intestines that may be due to microwave use.

There is a Japanese saying: "Where there is a front, there is a back. The larger the front, the larger the back." This means that things that may seem easy and enjoyable now may lead to larger, more costly problems later.

Macrobiotic educator Michio Kushi used to say, "Give your microwave to your best enemy or the military."

Air Pollution

The average person breathes two gallons of air per minute, which equals approximately 3,400 gallons of air each day.

Inhaling air pollution takes away at least one to two years of a typical human life.

It can cause effects as small as burning eyes and itchy throat, to as large as breathing problems and death.

Air pollution caused by waiting in traffic increases the chances of death caused due to heart attack.

The most hazardous pollutants are released from the air, more than water and land pollution combined.

Outdoor air pollution ranks in the top 10 killers on earth.

About 80% of lung diseases are caused by pollution from cars, buses, trucks, and other vehicles.

Detoxification

There are many methods of detoxification that can help remove toxins from the body.

The key is to open up the drainage routes that carry waste out of the body. They are called emunctories. The primary emunctories are the kidneys, liver, intestines, and lungs. Secondary elimination occurs through the skin, mucous membranes, nose, genitals, and joints.

Most symptoms that people take pills for are actually the body trying to detoxify. Taking pills may just cause suppression of the symptoms, but suppression works temporarily, and the body will find another exit. If all exits are closed, then toxins may end up in areas of less importance like fat cells, joints, gallbladder, uterus, or breasts, where the toxins may eventually cause further complications and disease.

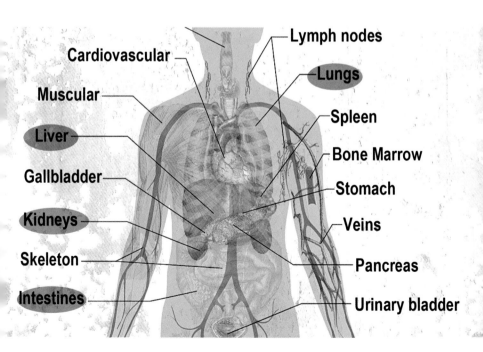

Tools to Detoxify

Fasting
Cleansing
Drinking clean water
Green, leafy vegetables
Seaweed
Lymphatic massage
Exercise
Colonics
Saunas

Biochemical methods: Herbs, vitamins, minerals.

Energetic methods: Laying on of hands, acupuncture, auricular medicine (ear acupuncture), homeopathy, qigong.

For 27 years I have been working with over ten thousand people on detoxifying. Some have a stronger detoxifying ability than others, but all can be healthier by avoiding toxins when we have a choice, and consciously working on detoxifying our bodies. You don't have to be a fanatic. Our bodies know how to detoxify, but remember that avoiding toxins is especially important for the fetus and children.

How to Detoxify

It is important to have your elimination organs functioning well, including your liver, kidneys, intestines, and skin.

Drink plenty of clean water, take saunas, do skin brushing, eat green leafy vegetables, consume probiotic foods or capsules.

Add healing spices such as cilantro, cinnamon, ginger, parsley, and turmeric

Have raw vegetables daily, or have juices such as apple, beet, celery, carrot, kale, and other dark leafy greens.

Add miso soup and seaweed to your diet.

Additional remedies to speed detoxification are use of a neti pot, castor oil pack, ginger compress.

Neti Pot or Sinus Irrigation

When we are exposed to air pollution, the hairs and mucous in our sinuses are the first line of defense.

Neti pots are typically made of metal, glass, ceramic, or plastic.

A simple yet effective technique is to pour saltwater solution into one nostril and let it run out through the other while the mouth is kept open to breathe, using gravity as an aid.

Plain water can be irritating to the sinuses, so it is best to use a saline solution.

Add ½ to 1 teaspoon of salt to each 16 ounces (two cups) of warm water. You can also add an additional ¼ teaspoon of baking soda per cup to the mixture. Use clean or purified water instead of tap water.

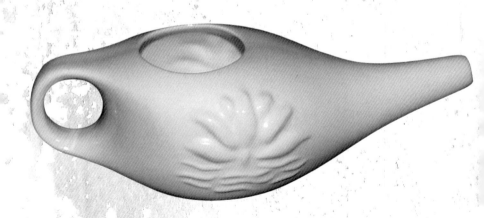

Castor Oil Pack

Castor oil has been used medicinally for thousands of years in Egypt, China, and India. In medieval Europe it was called palma Christi because the leaves resemble the hands of Christ.

It can be used topically for skin problems like dryness, rashes, hives, fungus, infections, boils, furuncles, liver spots (age spots), warts, and benign skin cancers.

If you want to improve detoxification I suggest making a castor oil pack or compress.

The most important place to place it is over the liver, under the right rib cage.

You can also place it over one of these areas.
- The kidneys in the small of the back
- Uterine fibroid or ovarian cysts
- Stomach, small or large intestines, if digestive issues bother you
- Lungs
- Painful joints

It is best not to place it over the heart.

Castor Oil Pack

1. Saturate a cloth with the oil, especially good is cotton or wool flannel. You could soak it in a one-quart mason jar to allow it to saturate.

2. Protect the area underneath you with plastic or a towel or sheet to protect the surface you'll be sitting or lying on.

3. Fold the cloth into three layers and place it on your skin. Put a hot pack (this is one time it's ok to use a microwave), hot water bottle, or heating pad over the cloth. Put plastic between the cloth and heat source as protection from the hot pack.

4. Keep the pack on for at least 20 minutes, and up to an hour. You can reuse the cloth many times. Keep it in a jar or sealed plastic bag, adding more oil each time you use it.

Ginger Compress

The benefits of a hot ginger compress are as follows.

- Dissolve stagnation
- Dissolve mucus and tension
- Melt blockages
- Stimulate circulation
- Stimulate energy flow

It also helps low back pain, and the liver, intestines, uterus, ovaries, lungs, and joints are other areas that will benefit as well.

The heat activity of the compress stimulates the blood and tissue circulation in the area being treated, which disperses the toxins, and then facilitates their excretion.

Since the kidneys tend to get cold easily, a ginger compress over the kidneys helps them flush out toxins and stones.

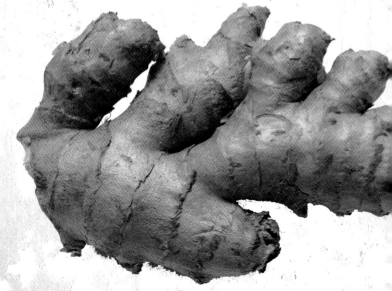

Ginger Compress

1. Bring a large pot of water to a boil. Meanwhile, grate enough ginger root to equal the size of a golf ball. When the water comes to a boil, reduce the heat to low. Then choose a method to proceed.

   - Faster than grating by hand, you can puree the ginger in water in a blender, then pour it into a strainer and lower it into the hot water.
   - Tie off the grated ginger in a cheesecloth, and place in water, keeping ends dry. Squeeze out until damp and not dripping.
   - Place it directly in the water and strain it into another pot.

2. Allow the ginger to steep five minutes.

3. Place a small towel into the ginger water, wring it out, and apply to the desired area on the body. Cover with another towel to hold in the heat. Change the cloth every two to three minutes as it starts to cool. Careful to keep it hot, but not enough to burn the skin.

4. Use two cloths, alternating them so that the skin does not cool between applications. Continue the applications for about 15 to 20 minutes until the skin has turned pink.

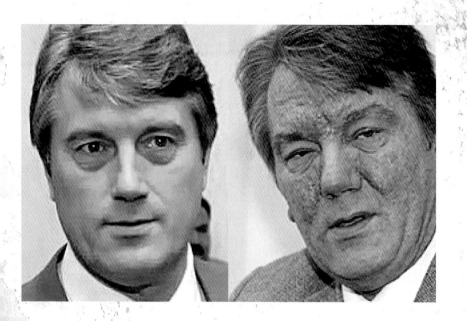

Can Toxins Make You Less Beautiful?

Viktor Yushchenko was poisoned by political
enemies in Russia with dioxin,
a common environmental toxin.

So if you still don't want to avoid toxins for all
the myriad health reasons, or the shortening of
your lifespan, then at least do it for vanity's sake!

Acknowledgments

I would like to thank all the people who have made this book possible.

My gratitude to Michio Kushi, Herman Aihara, and Steven Acuff for teaching the five elements and how they relate to diet and health.

Thanks to Shou-Yu Liang and Wen-Ching Wu for their teaching on medical qigong.

My gratitude to Connie Kroskin for designing what was a five-hour seminar into this beautiful book. Thanks for the artwork she contributed as well.

I am grateful for the careful editing by Elizabeth Binder while also helping to run a busy office.

Thanks to Caroline Danielson and Joni Wilson for their wonderful work on the final editing.

Many thanks to Nigel Yorwerth and Patricia Spadaro, my publishing consultants at publishingcoaches.com, for their expertise in helping bring this project to a new level, finding distribution in North America, and selling rights to my book worldwide.

Much love and gratitude to my wife, Paivi, for producing the beautiful pastel artwork for each element.

My thanks to all my patients and their organs for teaching me so much about how the body can heal. Gratitude to God and to all the invisible beings who assist me in my work.

About the Author

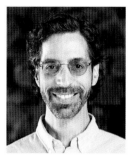

Warren King is a natural healer and educator who is passionate about teaching others to heal themselves. He was raised in a medical family and began his premedical studies at Cornell University. He later changed his focus to complementary medicine and alternative approaches to healing and went on to study Oriental medicine at the New England School of Acupuncture. Warren also attended the Kushi Institute to study healing through food with Michio Kushi. He continued his training in acupuncture as well as Chinese herbology under some of the finest Chinese medical doctors in the country at the New England School of Acupuncture as well as at the Midwest Center of Oriental Medicine in Chicago.

Warren has been a licensed acupuncturist for 27 years and has treated more than ten thousand patients with his unique multidisciplinary approach, constantly refining his knowledge, toolset, and intuitive skills to facilitate healing. Since most illnesses result from a combination of physical, mental, emotional, and spiritual causes, he believes that these must all be addressed for the best and most permanent results.

To find out more about Warren King, his books, online courses, membership site, and how to work with him one-on-one, visit warrenking.com.

Stay connected:

facebook.com/warrenkinghealth
instagram.com/warrenkinghealing
youtube.com/Warren King
twitter.com/IamWarrenKing
support@warrenking.com